THE RSI SURVIVAL GUIDE

THE RSI
SURVIVAL
GUIDE

THE RSI & OVERUSE INJURY
ASSOCIATION
OF THE ACT, INC

Authored by: RSI & Overuse Injury Association of the ACT, Canberra, Australia, 2.08 Griffin Centre, 20 Genge Street, Canberra City ACT 2601

Contact: admin@rsi.org.au

Editor: Ann Thomson

Contributors: Ann Thomson, Elizabeth Blackwell, Karen van den Broek, Kate Beckett, Kieu Huynh, Lia van den Bosch, Monique Williams, Robert Hawes, Shirley Pipitone, Steve Burns, Sue Woodward, Tegan Cruwys and many other people who generously contributed their ideas and experiences.

Copy Editors: Jane Thomson, Irene Turpie

First Published 2017

© The ACT RSI and Overuse Injury Association 2012

ISBN: 978-0-646-55208

TABLE OF CONTENTS

CHAPTER 1
INTRODUCTION

*I was 22 and working as a legal
secretary when I first felt pain in my
arms. I ignored it, thinking or hoping it
would go away, and continued to work
at my normal pace. I had recently
changed jobs and didn't want to cause
any problems. However, typing for six
or seven hours a day I soon realised the
pain was getting worse. It got to the
stage that I couldn't type more than a
few minutes at a time, and couldn't keep
up with the workload.*

There are lots of different names for RSI: occupational
overuse syndrome (OOS, complaints of the arms, neck and
shoulders (CANS), tendinopathy or tendinosis (for sports
injuries), Work-Related Upper-Limb Disorders (WRULD),
and even "cervicobrachial neurological syndrome"!

But whatever they're called, they hurt! Mostly, they hurt in
different parts of the upper body – carpal tunnel syndrome
in the wrists, epicondylitis in the elbows, and rotator cuff in
the shoulders. It's common for pain to start in one spot and
then spread to others.

*I was standing in front of a computer all
day, working as a pharmacist. Standing
all day tightens the muscles and
compresses the body and my working
conditions were very unergonomic. The
injury began to restrict my right arm
and shoulder and became so bad I had*

to take three months off work. I was
devastated when this happened.

How do I know if I have RSI?

These are some of the most common symptoms to look out for....

- burning, aching or shooting pain in small localised areas like fingertips, or larger areas like the forearm
- fatigue or lack of strength
- weakness in the hands or forearms to the extent that it's hard to do even simple things such as lifting a bag or shopping
- difficulty with normal activities like opening doors, chopping vegetables, turning on a tap
- chronically cold hands, particularly the fingertips

*I got RSI when I was working as a
source document operator, a job that
involved preparing documents to be put
onto microfiche film. A couple of months
after I started, the company won a
contract to transfer documents from a
large government department onto
microfiche. The majority of the
documents had staples that would
damage the lens if left in, so a co-worker
and myself spent an entire day picking
up documents and extracting staples
from them. I can't remember if it was
that afternoon or the following day that
the pain first occurred but I remember
how intense it was. It was like someone
was holding a blow-torch to my arm.
The pain was so bad that I couldn't
work.*

The first signs of an overuse injury are often soreness or tingling in the neck, arms, wrists, fingers or shoulders. These symptoms don't always happen straight away – you can experience them hours or even days after doing the activity that caused them.

Over time, what starts off as soreness and tingling can turn into a serious long term injury – so don't ignore it.

How do you get RSI?

You can get RSI by....

- doing something with your arms repeatedly for too long
- working with equipment that doesn't fit your body
- working too fast
- not having breaks
- holding your muscles in the same position for a long time
- not being trained in the safest way to carry out a task
- working for long hours
- not having enough variety in the type of work you do
- working with your arms above your shoulders
- working in cold conditions

Any or all of these things can lead to RSI, but the underlying cause common to all RSI-type conditions is damage to muscles and tendons (and the nerves that run through them) through repeated 'micro-trauma'.

What is micro-trauma? When you use your muscles, tiny tears sometimes happen in muscle tissue. The local area becomes inflamed for a short time as the body tries to repair the damage. Thickening and scar tissue form over the torn muscle tissue. At this stage, the area will hurt.

3

Normally, you'd rest for a while, your body would repair the damage and the pain would go away. But if you're not able to take a break – if you have to keep on working while your body is trying to heal the injury - further damage is caused instead. That leads to more inflammation, thickening, scar tissue and pain. Ultimately, you could develop a long-lasting overuse injury that will take years to get better.

It's actually possible to see this damage happening under a microscope, when changes happen in the structure of a tendon damaged by overuse. Bundles of collagen (a connective protein that allows flexibility and strength) that are normally tight and parallel instead look disorganised and discontinuous. You'd also see a decrease in fibre diameter and fibre loosening.

Not only are muscles damaged by RSI, but nerves are too. It's the compression of nerves that causes the tingling feelings people often get. Nerves run through muscles so if your muscle health is poor so is your nerve health. Damaged nerves **can** heal but the process is extremely slow.

TREATING RSI EARLY

Once RSI is established, it can be hard to cure and can have a major impact on your life. It can stop you from doing all kinds of things – working, playing a musical instrument, enjoying sports and doing basic housework for example. Some people with RSI eventually develop chronic pain that affects every aspect of their life. The good news, though, is that RSI can be cured in its early stages.

Myths about RSI

My wife was very understanding, as she had experienced RSI herself – so she could empathise with me. But I didn't speak to anyone else about it. There was such a stigma attached to RSI, and so much disbelief surrounding it, that I just didn't talk about my experience.

There are a lot of myths around RSI, and stigma too. This can be confusing and distressing if you suffer from it, and scary even if you don't.

1. RSI was invented in Australia in the 1980s

The *name* 'RSI' may have been coined in Australia in the 1980s, but the conditions associated with it have been known for hundreds of years. It was first described in the 1700s as a work-related condition by Italian physician, Bernadino Ramazzini. [1]

In 1870, there was an epidemic among British and French telegraphers, in 1911 among Morse key operators and in 1964 among Japanese keypunchers. In 1986, the *Australian National Occupational Health & Safety Commission* concluded that RSI was *not* new and *not* typically Australian. [2]

2. It's all in your mind

Arguments that RSI is psychological are based on the idea that people with RSI have anxiety and depression and *then* develop RSI. However, research has found that anxiety and depression are more likely to be *symptoms* of RSI than a cause. [3] As more research is conducted, more evidence of the physical causes of RSI is being published. Researchers have trained monkeys, rabbits and rats to do repetitive work for food – and they get RSI just like we do! [4]

3. RSI sufferers are just malingerers milking the compensation system

Some people think that people with RSI are pretending to be injured so they can get compensation. Not true. Many people with RSI don't apply for workers' compensation and just keep on working in pain. In fact, studies show that most people with symptoms of RSI have no intention of lodging a workers' compensation claim. People often decide not to claim because they're worried about being seen as a burden, taking time off work, or the effect that lodging a claim could have on their career, workload and working relationships.[5]

4. People who get RSI work in low-status, boring jobs

That might have been true in the past when most highly repetitive and/or forceful physical work was done by poorly-paid manual workers. But now that computers are widely used by white-collar workers and managers, people at all levels of the workforce get RSI. One study showed that RSI symptoms are found in 80% of salespeople, 81% of clerks, 86% of professionals and 78% of managers.

5. Only typists get RSI

RSI occurs in lots of industries and occupations, including journalists, butchers, hairdressers, musicians, carpenters and cleaners. Somewhat unexpectedly, the highest incidence of RSI occurs in meatworkers. You can also get RSI from leisure activities like golf, knitting, video games and playing a musical instrument.[6]

6. Only women get RSI

It's true that women are more likely than men to get RSI. However, the difference between male and female rates of RSI is small. In fact, the occupation with the highest incidence of RSI is – as we mentioned above - meatworkers, a field dominated by men.

The fact that women workers tend to do more work at home using the same muscle groups as those used at work could explain the higher rate of women with RSI.[7]

7. RSI only lasts a few weeks or months

A person can have RSI for just a short time if it's treated properly in the early stages, or for many years if it's not treated or diagnosed correctly in the beginning.[8]

8. To get better you need complete rest

Rest really helps with RSI, especially in the early stages. However, it's important to combine rest with exercise to help you recover and stay fit. Aerobic exercise, like walking or jogging, increases blood circulation to the injured area and helps it to heal. It also helps to counter depression.

9. No one gets RSI any more

The incidence of RSI is actually increasing. More than 60% of workers' compensation cases in the USA are for RSI and similar conditions.[9] In fact, RSI is very common - a recent article in the Lancet estimates that **5–10% of the general population** have an overuse injury that limits daily activity.

Research in Australia has revealed much higher figures within some professions. For example, 96.5% of a sample of Melbourne hairdressers reported a musculoskeletal disorder, a study of Australian academic staff and students found that 58% reported computer-related pain and a survey of ACT public servants found that 80% reported at least one symptom of overuse injury, with 23% of women and 12% of men reporting continuous pain in the upper body.

A survey of over 1000 Australian sonographers found that 90% reported a musculoskeletal disorder, with the main areas of pain in the shoulders, the upper back, arm and wrist. In all the studies quoted above, less than a quarter of the people affected had applied for workers' compensation.

CHAPTER 2
STAYING IN CONTROL AND MANAGING YOUR EMOTIONS

If I had to give advice to someone with RSI, it would be to try and retain control of your own life. It is difficult when you don't really understand what's going on, but remember that no one else can make the right decisions for you. Stay true to your instinct and follow it. Continue to believe in yourself and realise that your self-worth isn't wrapped up in what you can't do.

When you have RSI, and especially if you're in the workers' compensation system, it's easy to feel that you've lost control over many aspects of your life, such as your work, your health, your friendships and your family life.

In the end, I was in a lot of pain and was absolutely exhausted. I would go home after work and just lie down. It was getting to the point where I was buying TV dinners. I just couldn't face any more work.

So the focus behind much of this book is on how to take and keep control over your life. Having a sense of control over your own life is really important, both to managing daily life well and to help you in recovery.

I go to university full time and have two part-time jobs. I feel much more

independent than I have in the past,
even before my RSI. I can also
recognise when I need to ask for help or
take a break. It's much better to do this
than end up feeling that I have no
control over a situation.

To this end, we've included many hints, research findings, real life stories and technical advice. The main point here is, unless your RSI symptoms don't affect your ability to 'do what you've always done' at home, work, education or social situations, you're probably going to need to work on developing long-term strategies to deal with it. These strategies can help you regain and keep control over your life, even though you have a chronic condition. You can still aim to achieve the best emotional and physical health possible, and to live a fulfilling life.

The physical disability and ongoing pain of an overuse injury are also likely to affect your emotional well-being. You might grieve for the physical abilities that you've lost, the things you can't do any more and the changes in your way of life. You may feel emotions ranging from anger to apathy, hopelessness and depression.

You're not alone - depression or angry emotions are very common in people with RSI. But the good news is that these feelings might go away or become less overwhelming when you're supported by the right help and information.

When we talk to people with RSI, they say that it helps to let go of some of the fixed ideas they used to have, like "I have to devote myself to my work 110%", "I have to have a tidy house" or "only a meal I make from scratch is good enough for my family".

Letting go can be hard, but when you do, you're freeing yourself to make decisions that will help you get better. As one of our members pointed out:

You are the most important part of the
recovery process, not the ideas or
boundaries you've put in place.

Is it Normal to Feel Angry?

I didn't understand what was going on.
I had always been active and then I
couldn't work or take part in any sport
at all. I couldn't go to the movies or out
to dinner with friends either because I
couldn't sit or talk through the pain I
was experiencing. It was very
depressing and I was knocked sideways.
I had a very bad attitude in the
beginning too. I was angry and couldn't
believe how limited I was physically.

There was such a stigma attached to RSI
and so much disbelief surrounding it
that I just didn't talk about my
experience. I became very depressed
about what the future held and also
angry that I had been placed in that
situation.

Anger can be good – it can help you focus your energy on
getting your entitlements after your injury - but anger can
also become a destructive force holding you back. It takes a
lot of energy to stay angry, and that might be the energy you
need to deal with your RSI. It may help to stand back from
your anger and decide whether it's helping you or whether
it's actually stopping you from moving on.

If you need help to deal with your anger, get a referral to a
psychologist from your doctor.

Depression and RSI

There's no doubt that RSI can make you feel depressed. Studies have shown that people with musculoskeletal disorders (including RSI) have more than double the rate of depression of the rest of the population: at least 12% of people with these conditions are depressed.

> *"Anyone who begins each day awakened by pain is convinced that something is wrong with his or her body. But when a doctor can't find anything and family members grow suspicious, it is difficult not to doubt yourself or to drop into depression."*
>
> *- Fibromyalgia Network*

Psychologists think that depression has two main causes. The first is to do with the kind of person you are and the experiences you've had in your life. The second is to do with stress, and the kind of stress that's most likely to cause depression involves loss. This theory predicts that the more extreme your stress is and the longer it lasts, the more likely you are to develop depression.

Most people with an overuse injury go through not just one stressful event, but several. Many of these events involve some form of loss – such as the loss of good health and employment, for instance. Many people lose their social networks because they are closely connected with work. People can lose their ability to take part in sports and hobbies that make them feel good and connect them to other people.

Many people with overuse injuries lose their independence and suddenly find that they're dependent on family and friends to do simple things like hanging out the washing or cooking a meal. And of course, there's the loss of status that goes with losing your job and your income and suddenly becoming dependent on other people.

Furthermore, many of the stresses in the lives of people with work-related injuries go on for a long time – for instance, financial insecurity, involvement in the workers' compensation system and of course the pain itself. Most of us can recover from short-term stress, but stress that continues for a long time is more likely to cause depression.

There are two other important factors that make a person more likely to suffer from depression - and these are highly relevant to people who have RSI. The first is pain: studies show that the more pain a person is experiencing, the more likely they are to be depressed. This suggests that it's important to find a doctor who takes your pain seriously, one that you're able to work with to help you reduce your pain levels.

The second is helplessness. This is more likely to happen when a person with an overuse injury is in the workers' compensation system. Other people may be making important decisions for you and you may feel that you have little control over your own life, just at a time when it has become demanding and difficult.

Research has shown that situations like this tend to increase the likelihood of developing depression. There are two things that are important here – being in control, and **feeling** that you're in control. You'll benefit if you can increase the amount of control you have, and also if you can help yourself to **feel** that you have more control. Later on in this book, we have some suggestions about how to do this.

> *What helped me a lot – and I'm not the only one – was the active pursuit of mastery and meaning. I'd had to quit my job, but after this I found a way to volunteer from home for a cause that meant something to me. What might be even more important is that I started to explore and push the boundaries of what I could do physically. At first I made the mistake of pushing too hard – as if I*

*were getting revenge on my own body
for failing – but soon enough I learned
how to handle myself with kindness and
common sense. It made me friends with
my body again. Or, rather, it helped my
mind understand that my body had been
its friend all along.*

Having depression at the same time as a chronic disease
leads to a vicious cycle. The depression makes the chronic
disease worse, and the chronic disease makes the depression
worse. Part of the problem is that when you're depressed,
you're less likely to do the things that'll help you to get
better – such as getting exercise, sleeping well, keeping up
with treatments and eating good food. The other part is that
depression can harm your health – even if you're in good
shape to begin with.

Depression has a big impact on your life physically, not just
mentally as you'd expect. That's why it's really important
to get treatment as soon as possible for depression, as
you're more likely to recover from your overuse injury once
depression is treated successfully.

How do I Know if I have Depression?

The main symptom of depression –also the most obvious
one – is feeling miserable for at least two weeks at a time.
What most people don't realise is that anger is also a very
common symptom. Changes in sleep patterns, appetite or
weight – or in energy levels – can also be a sign. One very
important warning sign is if you've changed your routine to
accommodate your other symptoms (e.g. seeing your
friends less because you want to stay in bed).

What can I Do About it?

Depression is highly treatable– as many as 20% of people
experience it at some point in their lives. However, it's also

a very serious condition – one recent study found that it has a greater impact on your health than heart disease, diabetes or arthritis. So it's important to take your symptoms seriously.

The first step is to see your doctor, for two reasons. Firstly, depression can be a symptom of more serious hormonal problems (such as thyroid dysfunction) which can be ruled out through blood testing. Secondly, you need to get treatment for it.

What Happens in Therapy?

A lot of people don't like the idea of psychological treatment. TV shows about psychological therapy are all about dream analysis or discussing your troubled childhood – but that's not what happens in modern psychology.

Two modern methods of psychological therapy that work pretty well for depression are Cognitive Behavioural Therapy (CBT) and Interpersonal Therapy – and most therapists in Australia have some background in these.

CBT involves looking at and questioning the thoughts and behaviours that keep you depressed, as well as learning to control negative thinking. Interpersonal therapy focuses on better ways of handling relationships and stress, and learning how to think about and manage situations that trigger depression.

Some psychologists specialise in treating people with chronic pain and can teach you how to manage your pain in a structured way. If you try therapy and don't like it, try another therapist – there are a lot of different approaches out there.

Some alternative therapies for depression (supported by good scientific evidence) involve the herb St John's wort and omega-3 fish oils (which seem to help prevent depression). There's also some evidence for the benefits of acupuncture, massage therapy, relaxation, folate, and yoga breathing exercises.

What about Anti-Depressants?

Medications are sometimes a good option for treating depression in the short-term. SSRIs are the most commonly prescribed, as they have the fewest side effects. However, drug treatments without psychotherapy don't work in the long term because the depression comes back. On top of this, about 30% of people don't respond to drug treatment at all, whereas about 90% of people report some benefit from a course of psychotherapy.

Preventing Depression when you have RSI

- Keep up your social life, even if you have to find new ways of socialising with your friends. Research shows that you're a lot less likely to get depression if you have an active social life.
- Get some exercise. Exercise is an effective method of preventing *and treating* depression. It's also one of the best ways to help you recover from RSI, so make time to do something that doesn't make your condition worse - like brisk walking.
- If you're involved in a medico-legal dispute, try to distance yourself mentally from the hurtful reports and other difficulties that arise.
  Try not to see these as a personal attack – that's just how the system works.
- Meaningful volunteer work can be very fulfilling, and there are satisfying positions available where you won't need to use your arms.
- Try to see obstacles as challenges you can solve – don't just give up.

15

- Think about what you'll need help with – you might need to let go of some independence to minimise your pain.

Challenge Negative Self-Talk

Self-talk is what you say **to** yourself *about* yourself. Everyone does it, and it affects how you feel every day. After an injury, you might start thinking differently about yourself, for example: "I will never be able to cope with this", "It's not fair", "I can't do anything about this pain", "They're all out to wreck my life."

To have more control over your life, it helps if you become aware of your self-talk, recognise repetitive negative thoughts and learn how to challenge them. Negative thoughts can become a habit if you let them.

Next time you think something bad about yourself or something you're trying to do, write it down, and then read it back and ask yourself:

- Is this really true or am I exaggerating?
- Is this thought helping me to feel better about myself or worse?
- How can I change this thought to something more positive and realistic?

You can challenge negative thoughts by changing each one to a more positive – and realistic – alternative. By doing this, you're taking control and helping yourself feel good.

Challenge yourself when you find yourself making statements about 'everyone' and 'everything' and using words like 'always' and 'never'. Yes, we recognise that systems or organisations are often at fault. But it's important not to let yourself start seeing things in terms of black and white. Reality is rarely like that.

Whether things are running smoothly or not, reality has many shades of grey. If you find yourself saying to yourself "this is hopeless", stop and ask yourself 'Why can't I do this? Is there another direction I can take?'

Try to find more helpful ways of talking to yourself about the situation. It may not be as bad as you think it is. For example, if you're feeling depressed and your arms hurt, it can be hard to keep up with friends. You might be thinking to yourself "What's the point of seeing people? I can't cook and I've got nothing to talk about anyway."

So maybe you can answer yourself, "I can arrange to meet my friends at a café and just chat as I always have. They love me and they'll understand." Now you're putting yourself back in control. You're reminding yourself that the situation isn't hopeless, and you can still do things you'll enjoy.

Try talking to yourself as you would to a good friend. You have an illness and it's not your fault. You need comfort and understanding. You deserve care –including from yourself – when you're feeling ill. Tell your friends and family how they can help. You need people who'll listen and be in your corner. A good support group can be helpful too.

Take Back Control

When you have RSI, you might feel your life is out of your control. But in fact you **do** have some choices and you can make decisions based on these choices.

When the whole situation seems overwhelming, you might start thinking in black and white – everything is either good or bad. You might let other people control what happens in your life, like family matters, work and your compensation claim. Sometimes because you feel you don't have control over your situation, you might start to feel worthless and useless. But if you recognise this negative cycle you can change it!

Know Your Rights

One of the best things you can do is to know your rights. Everyone has rights and these rights are important. You have the right to speak up for yourself, to be treated fairly and to be treated with respect. You have the right to be treated in this way by everyone you encounter – family, friends, doctors, case-managers and employers.

Taking back responsibility for your own life is liberating, but it may take time. You might want to start with small decisions –like deciding how to spend your day or making a budget. That might not sound like much – but it's important to keep making decisions, however small, so you feel in charge of your daily life.

Even if you stand up for yourself, there's no guarantee that you'll get what you want every time. You're probably going to be dealing with people who have financial interests at stake, fixed opinions, or are used to getting their own way by behaving dishonestly or aggressively. But at least you can walk away knowing that you acted in a way that respects yourself and others.

Standing up for yourself – and learning to talk to yourself positively and sympathetically – will help you feel better in the long run!

Stress and RSI

What Is Stress?
We hear about 'stress' a lot. People usually say they're stressed when they feel they can't cope with the demands placed on them, and when they feel tense or uncomfortable. **Stress is an emotion you experience when you feel that you don't have the resources to deal with a particular situation**.

When we experience a stressful situation, our bodies undergo what's called 'the stress response' – changes that get the body ready for action. These include an increased heart rate, increased respiration, muscle tension and feeling alert.

Why do we get stressed?

Why does the 'stress response' make us get tense and agitated right when we need to concentrate the most?

In our evolutionary past, we didn't have to deal with exams, traffic and losing our job. Instead, we had to cope with predators, fire, flood, earthquake, and so on. To survive, early humans could either *fight* the danger or *flee* from it. So our stress response gets us ready for a burst of physical energy – fight or run.

These days that's not so useful. The things that stress modern humans the most in the developed world are financial strain, relationships and problems at work. You can't solve that kind of problem by physically fighting or running away.

Another thing about modern stress is that it's often *chronic*. Instead of an urgent threat to your life that goes away pretty quickly one way or another, modern stress goes on and on. Because of this, your body's stress response is maintained over long periods, causing a range of health problems.

What causes stress?

Anything that you see as a threat – physically, emotionally or socially – can be stressful. You can be stressed out by bad things you *expect* to happen as well as what's already happened, and that's where RSI can be extremely stressful.

When you have RSI, you can feel worried about your health and your future. It's also very stressful to feel like you don't have much control over what happens to you. If you're on workers' compensation, you probably feel like you have much less control over your life than you did before.

Lots of things can be stressful, but it's only when you see them as bad that they have an effect on your health. A wedding can be pretty stressful but it doesn't usually make you ill. So the way you think about what's happening matters when you're trying to manage your stress. Negative thoughts can exaggerate your problems and make you underestimate how well you can cope with them.

Workplace stress and muscle health

Not only is having RSI pretty stressful, other stresses at work can actually contribute to RSI.

According to psychologist Dr Bob Montgomery, "the simple major determinant of work-related stress is how much say you have in how you do your job. The less say you have – particularly if demands are put on you – the higher your stress rate, the poorer your health."

Are overuse injuries related to stress? In a recent paper published in the *American Journal of Industrial Medicine*, three American researchers looked at the connections between stress and RSI. The authors stated there is plenty of evidence about the role of workplace stress in both causing overuse injuries and making them worse.

How does workplace stress contribute to overuse injury? The paper suggested a number of ways that stress might contribute. According to the research, when people are stressed, they move differently, become stiffer, stay in the same position for longer, tend not to relax as quickly after a task is finished and have more tense muscles.

Other studies have measured muscle tension in workers and have found that levels are much higher when people are stressed at work. For example, a Finnish study measured muscle tension in home helpers, bank clerks and nurses, focusing particularly on shoulder and neck muscles.

Other research suggests that stress affects breathing and this is a factor in overuse injury. This works in two ways. Firstly, people who are stressed often breathe in the upper chest rather than using their diaphragm. This recruits muscles in the neck and shoulder area and imposes stress on the whole neck and shoulder region.

Secondly, people who are stressed often over-breathe or hyperventilate. This basically means breathing in more oxygen than you need. According to this research, hyperventilation triggers a chain of reactions in your body including constriction of blood vessels, a decrease in the oxygenation of muscle tissue and a build-up of metabolites (by-products of muscle activity). Obviously, all three of these will contribute to poor muscle health.

People with RSI suffer from a number of very significant stressors. Loss of health, job and income, chronic pain and an uncertain future can all cause a lot of stress. Additionally, people claiming workers' compensation often lose control over their treatment – and rehabilitation programs may then take control over the pace of their return to work. With all these stressors affecting people with RSI, it's important to realise that there are ways to counter stress and deal with the demands placed on you.

What can I do to counter stress?

There are quite a few things you can do to help you cope with the stresses that can go with having an overuse injury. Exercise is a great way to reduce the impact that stress has on you, both immediately and in the longer term. Exercise also has protective effects: people who exercise regularly respond better and have fewer health consequences following a significant life stressor. Additionally, exercise is a good way to hasten your recovery from overuse injury as the increased circulation speeds healing. Try an aerobic exercise you'll enjoy, whether it's brisk walking or dancing. Step back from anything that strains your affected muscles.

Another factor that can help you cope better is your social support network. People with more close contacts (and anyone who you feel comfortable sharing personal information with counts) suffer less anxiety and depression.

People with overuse injuries often feel very isolated, and it's easy to see how pain can prevent you from being a social butterfly. But maintaining and expanding your social network is something you can do if you decide to make it a goal. Joining community organisations, such as social, religious, special interest, or self-help groups is a good place to start, as the people you meet will already have something in common with you!

Another suggestion is to volunteer your time – many organisations offer positions which do not require writing or computing. You'll not only meet new people but feel really good about it too! (Visit www.govolunteer.com.au for a searchable database of volunteer jobs in your area.)

Remember, the easiest way to maintain social support is to make the effort to stay in contact. If your friends don't ring you, ring them – you'll both live longer for it!

Another strategy that can help is to change how you approach problems. Being optimistic and organised, focusing on problem solving, and maintaining a sense of personal control will make a huge difference to how stressed you feel and reduce the impact of stress on your health.

One of the best ways to maintain a sense of personal control is to get as much *information* as you can – about your condition, treatment options and management techniques. For example, it's been found that simply providing hospital patients with more information reduces their use of medication, length of hospital stay and post-operative pain, and also speeds up their overall recovery. Preparation for stressful events, both by gaining information and planning solutions, improves your coping skills when under stress.

Relaxation

Learning to relax is probably one of the most important skills you can learn to help you manage RSI – and it may also help you to recover.

By 'relaxing', we mean knowing what your body feels like when muscles are tense and then being able to loosen those muscles, letting them go so that they are fully relaxed.

Tight muscles when you're doing something mean that your body has to work harder to get the job done and this puts more strain on your injury. For example, imagine you have your shoulders tightly scrunched while you're typing. This could be because you're feeling worried and tense about something or it could just be your habitual way of working. Researchers can measure how hard muscles work and have found that when people are stressed, their muscles work much harder to do the same job compared to when they are working normally.

So those tight shoulders are making you work a lot harder to achieve the same result. They're not doing you a favour! And that tightness might persist through the day, even when you're not working. That's why becoming aware of how to relax your muscles is really important.

One of the simplest techniques to achieve relaxation is to lengthen the outbreath, that is, breathe out for longer than you breathe in. Pushing more oxygen out of your body physically slows the breathing and heart rate, which means there's less blood pumping to your muscles, reducing tension.

Try sitting in a comfortable position and breathing in slightly deeper than you usually would for 3 counts, and breathing out for 4. You'll feel your heart rate slow and your muscles begin to relax. This technique can require a bit of practice, and it might help to follow a guided relaxation app or CD.

Another useful technique for stress and pain management is 'progressive muscle relaxation'. This method targets the muscle tension that usually accompanies chronic pain and stress.

The idea of this method is to purposely tense different parts of the body and then release them. If you experience tension in your neck and shoulders, start by trying this method with your feet and hands. As an experiment, try sitting or lying in a comfortable position and tensing the muscles in your feet. Notice the tension and effort it requires to do this. When you're ready, relax your feet. Notice that your feet feel less heavy, and it's less of an effort to hold this relaxed position.

Now you can move up your body, tensing and relaxing your lower legs, upper legs, pelvic area, lower back, stomach, upper back, hands, arms, shoulders, neck and head. Always tense and relax in the same order (whichever one you choose), as this will help to form a useful mental script you can follow any time you want.

Following a voiced guide through a CD or app can be very helpful. If tensing a particular area is painful, instead just direct your mental attention to that part of the body and then relax it.

The best part about these two methods is that they actually work! A five-year follow-up study of participants suffering from chronic musculoskeletal pain found that if participants continued to perform relaxation breathing techniques, their pain ratings decreased – and stayed that way. In addition to being more cost-effective, less difficult to incorporate into daily life, and easier to manage than other forms of pain management, participants rated themselves as happier as well.[10]

If you'd like to learn in a class, yoga relaxation groups can be very helpful. There are also quite a few helpful guided relaxation apps you can download to your smartphone, for example, Calm, Buddhify, and Headspace.

When you don't have much time, you can do a short guided meditation; for example, you can imagine a 'shower of relaxation' progressively soothing your head, neck, shoulders, arms, chest, abdomen and legs – and this only takes less than a minute.

In short, learning the skill of muscle relaxation can

- Lessen stress
- Help you get to sleep
- Decrease the amount of effort you use to achieve tasks
- Help you to heal
- Help you to manage anxiety
- Decrease pain levels

When Someone Close to you has RSI

If you're a partner or close family member of someone who has RSI, this section is for you.

Watching someone you love deal with pain and frustration can be very hard. You probably don't know exactly what you can do to help and they might not be able to tell you what they need from you. This is going to put extra pressure on your relationship.

For instance, your partner might become more dependent on you physically- but shut you out emotionally. You might feel that with all the focus on your partner's needs, your own needs aren't being met. The situation might feel like a big burden on your shoulders. You know you need to be there for your partner – but it can all seem very one-sided. Unless you've been through a similar situation yourself, you probably won't know what your partner's going through, or how to help them. It's normal.

Work together!

> *I'd had RSI for about six years when my partner and I decided we wanted to have a child. At that time, in 2000, I was working full-time and attending regular treatments to manage the pain. It was a difficult decision because we were both nervous about the kind of impact pregnancy and looking after a baby would have on my body... Throughout the pregnancy there was a lot to think about, and organisation was very important. My partner and I had to anticipate the problems that might arise and work out how we would cope so we gathered as much information as we could. We read everything we could find, and spoke to other people with RSI who'd had children to learn how they coped. We also found community resources and services we could use, such as community nurses.*

When one partner in a relationship is chronically ill, it's a shared issue - one that needs to be dealt with together. It's important to face the challenges as a team and, together, figure out how you as a couple will cope. Too often couples go off into their own little corners, trying to manage as best they can on their own. A better approach is to try to solve the problems together.

It's not their fault

Don't make your partner feel guilty for being ill. They didn't ask to get RSI, and if they could get better, they definitely would! It's easy to start resenting the difficulties that living with chronic illness brings into your life, but try not to let bitterness creep into your relationship. It can be really destructive.

Remember the person

Your partner is special to you. Don't let the illness make you forget that. The pressures of living with someone who's chronically ill can make you start to see them as a nuisance or a burden. But don't give in to this temptation. Remember how much your partner has added to your life through the years, and hold onto hope for better times in years to come.

Be flexible

Chronically ill people often have good days and bad days. So sometimes it's hard for you as their partner to switch gears from one day to the next. When you see your partner up and about, capable and on top of things one day – and the next, unable to manage even simple tasks, it can be very frustrating. If you're confused by what's going on, ask your partner what kind of day they're having. This can help you figure out what to expect from him or her.

> *It was very distressing for my partner as well, to see the change in me and the ultimate restrictions on his lifestyle. My RSI had repercussions for both of us, but he was wonderful, and did everything he could to help me recover. He still does all the heavy housework for me and will even iron when he has to! I am very lucky in having such a supportive husband and I couldn't have managed without him.*

Make a backup plan

When you're living with someone with a chronic illness, life is unpredictable. So when you plan to go somewhere or do something with your partner, have Plan A, B, and even C ready to go! If the first plan doesn't work out, not to worry – you've got it covered.

Keep up your own hobbies and interests

You need to keep up your own hobbies and interests separate from your chronically ill partner. If you don't allow yourself time off from the responsibility of living with, or caring for, a chronically ill person, you're likely to burn out. Try to do something special for yourself – whether it's for a couple of hours or a full weekend getaway. While you're taking time out, find someone who can be on call for your partner if a problem or crisis comes up. Give yourself a break!

Your partner isn't their illness

If you're angry about the effect of your partner's illness on your life, don't take your anger out on them. It's normal to feel angry, depressed, sad, frustrated and scared when you're living with a chronically ill person. Give yourself permission to grieve for what you've lost in your lives, separately and together. Grieving together as a couple can be a very healing thing. Go to a counsellor if you need help working through your grief.

Be supportive, but don't try to fix things

If your partner is struggling with their health, don't try to 'fix' them. You can't. Try instead to be a good listener, and offer comfort and compassion. You might say something helpful and encouraging like, "I'm sorry you're struggling. You've been through a lot. We'll make it through this together." Emotional support like this can really help lift your partner's spirits!

My partner is very important to me; he has been so accommodating and supportive. There has always been the extra pressure, and the physical load on him has been much greater. From the beginning there have been certain things I couldn't do, such as bathing our daughter or chopping vegetables. We have different roles, and our daughter has learnt this too. She knows that

Mummy can't play certain games that
Daddy can, and she knows that Mummy
gives hugs on the floor and Daddy
doesn't.

Live a balanced life
It can be tempting to find lots of things to do and places to
be so that you don't have to be constantly around your
partner's pain. But if you do, it will probably leave your
partner feeling neglected, depressed and hurt. Make sure
you spend special time with your partner, even if it's just
watching a video together or talking. Enjoy the simple
things in life together.

Try to be positive and optimistic
Try to be as positive and optimistic as much as possible, for
yourself and for your partner. It generally helps to try to
look on the bright side, if you can – but we know that can
be easier to say than to do.

Remember that real life is not perfect
Life is not perfect and never will be. You probably didn't
plan to spend your life with someone who has a chronic
illness – but then, your relationship is for better or for
worse, richer or poorer, in sickness and in health. Now's
your chance to show how steadfast you can be.

Help make your home somewhere your partner can safely express their feelings
Your partner desperately needs a nurturing, safe place to
express their feelings about the illness, without feeling
threatened, constrained or condemned. So try to make your
home that kind of place.

Divorce won't solve your problems
Your partner's illness affects your entire family. But it's
NOT their fault. It's not your fault either - it just is. You
might see divorce as a way to escape the situation – but in
reality, you're probably just going to swap one set of

problems for another. Instead, try to work through challenges together as a couple, learning and growing through them instead of just running away.

Above all else, never lose hope!

If you feel you're at the end of your rope and are just hanging on, then - hang on! Just when you think you can't take it anymore, things will most likely start to get better. People with chronic illness often have ups and downs in their health so keep hoping and believing that life will be better in the future – and it probably will.

Additional Resources

Beyond Blue provides information on depression. They can send out information kits and booklets and refer you to doctors and psychologists. They have lots of useful fact sheets including ones on help for depression, anxiety-related disorders, and chronic physical illness and depression.

Call their **Info Line** on **1300 224 636** or visit their website: www.beyondblue.com.au

Lifeline is a 24-hour counselling service staffed by trained volunteers.
Phone: **13 11 14**

CHAPTER 3
MANAGING YOUR TREATMENT

*The best advice I could give to anyone
with newly diagnosed RSI is to make
sure you have a good doctor – one who
is prepared to understand your
condition and help 100%. If not, find
someone else.*

Choosing a Doctor

Your doctor can be a powerful source of support and
information throughout your RSI journey. You don't need
to have the perfect GP – but you do need one that's good
enough.

Try to find a doctor who has:

- a caring and empathic attitude
- knowledge of overuse injuries and experience in
  treating them
- the ability to put you in contact with good
  specialists
- some knowledge of your work life or is willing to
  learn
- a willingness to fill in forms and support you if
  you're in the compensation system

If your doctor doesn't have these qualities, think about
changing doctors. You can always stay with your current
GP for most things, but get them to refer you to someone
more knowledgeable for your RSI – perhaps another GP or

a specialist. Feel free to look around until you find a doctor who meets your needs.

This isn't 'doctor-shopping' – it's the logical thing to do when you value your health and you need to find the best treatment.

On your first visit to a new doctor, try asking these questions:

- how do you feel about treating this condition (RSI)?
- are you willing to deal with my insurance company?

Since there's no treatment for RSI that works for everyone, your doctor will have to try out different treatments to see what will work for you. There is no magic bullet. But you can help your doctor by reading up on the research on RSI and sharing it with them.

How you feel about the relationship with your doctor is vital to your treatment. If you're not comfortable with the doctor or you feel they don't care enough about your condition, try another doctor. If you feel rushed or intimidated while you're talking to them, then you're probably not going to be able to talk to them fully about your symptoms or ask the questions you need to. You need to feel at ease with your doctor for him or her to really support you through this.

Specialists

RSI can affect your neck, shoulders, forearms, and hands, as well as blood circulation, nerves and muscles. So which specialist should you go to? Here are some suggestions:

- neurologists (the nervous system)
- rheumatologists (muscles and joints)
- occupational physicians (work-related injuries)
- sports medicine specialists

Although sports medicine specialists are often very experienced in treating overuse injuries in athletes, their patients are generally fit and in top physical condition. If that doesn't sound like you, you might find the treatments they prescribe aren't as effective for your condition. They're still worth trying though.

Will my Doctor be my Advocate?

People with RSI need a doctor who'll be available for them over the long haul, and who is willing to provide relevant evidence and reports if required. Your doctor may need to provide frequent medical reports to people and organisations such as your employer, insurance company, rehabilitation provider and solicitor. Centrelink may also be involved.

So your doctor needs to be willing to do all this, and act as your advocate in negotiations about any workplace redesign you might need to help in your return to work. If you have a workers' compensation case, your doctor will need to understand the workers' compensation system, be willing to be your advocate and be able to resist pressure.

Should I See a Psychologist or a Psychiatrist?

Sometimes your doctor might refer you to a psychologist or psychiatrist, or suggest you see one. You might be worried that these specialists will look for a psychological cause for your injury, but they usually won't.

Some psychologists and psychiatrists are experts in pain management and can help you deal with the very real pain of RSI. They might also explore ways of coping with your injury, help you deal with the grief and emotional effects of your disability and support you in moving on with your life.

Self-Education

When people suffering from a chronic illness take an active part in managing their own condition, it can help them feel in charge and improve their health.

So it's worth learning as much as you can about your condition and treatment options – for instance by reading about it, talking to other people with RSI, and searching the internet.

A great source of information about treatments that work is the Cochrane Collaboration – an association involving thousands of researchers, medical practitioners and consumers from around the globe.

For more information, or to find some easy-to-read information about your own healthcare options, visit the Cochrane Database via the website: www.cochrane.org or for summaries with an Australian slant visit: www.healthdirect.gov.au.

And don't forget our website and newsletter!

Stigma

Unfortunately, there can be a stigma attached to having RSI, so you might not feel like talking to people about it. But how can you get help and support if you don't? Some ideas for dealing with stigma are:

- Make sure it doesn't get to you and create doubt and shame. If you feel this is happening, get help.
- Don't stay with any therapist who makes you feel bad about your condition. There are plenty of good people around who won't do that.
- Don't isolate yourself to avoid possible stigma. It's really important for your mental health to stay in touch with friends and family.
- You have a choice about who to talk to about your illness and how much you say. If you do decide to

talk about how you feel, try to be frank but brief: "Sorry, I wasn't up to cooking today. Let's go to a coffee shop!"

- Don't apologise too much – your condition is a fact that you can't do a lot about. Being apologetic will not help your relationships or make you feel good.

If you'd like to read more, there is a website for people with invisible illnesses with lots of ideas for what to say, how to manage at work and how other people can be more helpful. Take a look at: https://www.kaleidoscopefightinglupus.org/invisible-illness-but-you-look-so-good/

Write it Down!

I found one thing I could do which really helped me with my doctor. I got my husband to follow me around for a day and take notes about everything I could and couldn't do. My husband typed up the report and I took it to the doctor. I found that my doctor really hadn't understood the extent of the problem until I did this.

It often helps if you make an effort to notice and record how your pain affects you every day. How does it affect your work, leisure activities, sleep patterns, ability to walk, sit, drive and so on? Notice what makes your pain better or worse - for example, do you feel better or worse after exercise? Better in the morning or at night? It's worth writing down all of this for your doctor, including what you can and can't do.

Keep a file containing your personal medical information. It should have copies of reports and tests, and a record of medications taken (especially if they had any ill-effects).

Caring for your health is a responsibility that you share with your doctor.

If you're seeing a new doctor, write a summary of your medical history and take it with you on your first visit. Ideally it should be about a page long. Have two copies, one for the doctor and one for your file at home. It's a good way to make sure you don't forget to mention something important.

For the same reason, write a list of questions you want to ask about your condition and treatments. A friend or family member might be able to help with the writing involved. Don't be embarrassed about referring to the list while you're at the doctor – you'll be helping both yourself and your doctor.

You could take a partner, relative or close friend with you. This can be really helpful when you're anxious, upset, in too much pain to listen well, or you can't take notes. Ask questions – if you don't understand something the doctor says, ask them to explain again in a way you do understand.

Spare a thought for the doctor, though, and don't offload everything at once. Focus on just a few issues for each visit: for instance, you might say something like "Things are still really hard generally, but today I really wanted to ask you about…"

Keeping a Pain Diary

A pain diary is where you keep a record of your pain and how it changes from day-to-day, how you feel about it, what makes you feel better and what makes you feel worse.

Yes, maybe it sounds a bit miserable, but it can be really helpful in lots of ways. For instance, it can help you see connections between your pain and things that happen or that you do – so it helps you get more control over your pain in the long term. By keeping an eye on what happens over the weeks and months, you can see whether therapies are working or not and how pain might be affecting your moods.

Don't be afraid that focusing on your pain will make you depressed. According to Deborah Barrett, the author of 'Pain Tracking', "You need to know exactly what you're facing and not live with an account based on hopes or fears. Objective data enables you to assess the areas needed for improvement and communicate more effectively with healthcare professionals." In other words, a pain diary puts you in command and lets you see what's really happening, rather than just living day to day.

Another plus is that it will help you give a more accurate picture to your doctor of what you're experiencing. Usually, if we see the doctor on a "good" day, we'll probably tell them that things are not too bad. But if you've been keeping a pain diary, you'll be able to give the doctor a more accurate picture because you'll know what it was like yesterday, and last week. It's even better if you've rated your pain on a numerical scale (see below). Since that's how medical professionals usually assess pain, they'll know exactly what you mean.

Moreover, a pain diary will help you notice what therapies are working for you – and what isn't working. One member said, "I started to notice that there was a real pattern of bad headaches after each massage session. My therapist was able to adjust his techniques so this didn't happen." Another member says "I had a great relationship with a particular therapist. We had lots of interests in common and I really used to enjoy our chats. But my pain diary showed that the therapy simply was not working and was basically a waste of my time and money."

A pain diary can guide you in a new, more helpful direction. "After keeping a pain diary, I realised I had always been too optimistic about my RSI," says one of our members. "It made me see that I needed to adapt what I was doing and get more help from my family. I needed to rethink my priorities as well."

But how can you keep a diary if your RSI makes it hard to write, as it often does? One way is just to make really brief notes. For instance, you could keep a record of your pain using a numerical scale from 1 to 10, where 1 is no pain at all and 10 is the most extreme pain you can imagine. So all you have to write is a number. To show where the pain is, you can make up your own shorthand like, "W" for wrist, "RS" for right shoulder and so on.

A pain diary can record more than where the pain is and how much it hurts. 'Pain Tracking' author Deborah Barrett suggests you might want to record some of the following:

- your overall pain experience (whether your pain feels all-consuming or manageable, in spite of how strong it is)
- how tired you are
- your energy level
- your mood, and
- your overall well-being.

You could make a note of more positive measures of how things are going for you, like your social life or how well you coped with your pain. It's also a good idea to make a note about how well you sleep – but the main thing is to record what matters to you!

You can get some good ideas for pain diaries from the internet and you can find different templates online.

It's a good idea to set a regular time of day for filling in your pain diary so you don't forget.

> *I like to fill in my diary at the end of the day and keep it beside my bed with a pen. It's something I make myself do before I go to bed and then I like to have a look at it when I wake up to help me make decisions about my day.*

In short, a pain diary can really help you manage your pain, communicate about it clearly and focus on treatments that really work.

Surgery

If surgery is recommended, it's vital that you get a second opinion. Read as much as you can about the operation and talk to other people who've had it if you can. Find out about the surgeon's reputation for the particular operation suggested. Ask them directly about:

- their success rate
- possible side effects or complications
- how long you will be out of action
- how many times they have performed the procedure recently.

If a doctor prescribes drugs, tests or x-rays, make sure that they explain what the potential risks, benefits and side-effects are. Ask about alternatives that may be less expensive, less risky, or less uncomfortable.

If you want to know more about drugs, talk to your pharmacist. Anti-inflammatory medications are often prescribed for RSI but their side-effects can be severe, including gastro-intestinal bleeding and heart problems – especially if you're older. Your pharmacist may be able to suggest a safer alternative. Make sure to tell your pharmacist about any other medicines you're on, for your own safety.

The Treatment Wilderness

In 1991 three researchers from the University of Sydney published a study based on interviews with fifty-two women workers with RSI from two workplaces. A strong theme that emerged from the interviews was that most of the women were trying to manage their condition in 'a treatment wilderness'.

When they were first diagnosed, the women were recommended one treatment after another, none of which seemed to work. As time went on and they became desperate to get well and get back to work, they tried more and more treatments, which mostly still didn't work.

> *The women often exhausted their own resources in finding a helpful and sympathetic doctor... (trying) avenues for new and untried therapies in the hope that there was a practitioner somewhere who would both believe and help them. A large part of their lives became absorbed in seeking advice and care from medical and health professionals who were either as bewildered as they – or in the case of some specialists – frankly sceptical. (There was) a bewildering array of treatments offered to the women, none of which were permanently effective, a very few of which provided temporary relief and most of which either exacerbated the problem or had no effect.[11]*

In 1999, a UK researcher, Hilary Arksey, published the results of her interviews with people with RSI. Their experiences were similar:

> *The first orthopaedic surgeon I saw had no idea what I was talking about, did not take the problem seriously and had only one suggestion: steroid injections. This was so painful and entirely without beneficial effect that I cancelled my subsequent appointment.*

*The treatment I was advised to
undertake – physiotherapy – could have
done more damage had I not decided to
stop at an early stage.* [12]

The interviewees talked about their frustration and
dissatisfaction with the world of medicine. Many of them
were on a medical merry-go-round of interviews with
different specialists and trying out different treatments.

So is it different in Australia today? It seems not. From
interviews we did recently, it's obvious that people with
RSI are still having very similar experiences today:

*I tried everything – osteopathy,
chiropractic, acupuncture, and
homeopathy. I kept thinking that if only I
do this or this it will get better, someone
will fix me. I was searching for some
treatment or therapy to fix my RSI but
nothing helped.*

*I tried every treatment recommended to
me. I had acupuncture and did Pilates
twice a week, saw an osteopath every
fortnight and had a massage once a
week. I was worn out from the constant
appointments. My life centred around
my injury.*

*I was seeing a physiotherapist,
specialists and my GP and I tried
acupuncture, Bowen therapy and
massage – nothing worked.*

How do I Find a Treatment that Works?

Here are a few ideas on how to figure out which treatments
work for you:

- limit the number of treatments you have at the same time – you need to be able to see what's helping you and what isn't
- give each type of treatment a good try, but don't stay with something that isn't working (six to eight weeks is generally enough time for most treatments to show some sort of result)
- talk to therapists about expected pain levels
- keep in touch with research
- talk to other people with RSI who are at a similar stage of the condition
- keep track of pain and disability, and things that might affect them
- get back to your GP/specialist regularly
- time treatments carefully (e.g. massage *after* gym work, not immediately before)
- find a GP who treats many people with RSI

Unfortunately, there's still no treatment with a really strong evidence base for overuse injuries because the research that's available isn't comprehensive enough to show what works. A group of Scandinavian researchers analysed all the studies they could find that looked at overuse injury treatment, and concluded that "no strong evidence was found for the effectiveness of any of the treatment options," and that "little was known about the effectiveness of conservative treatment options for repetitive strain injury." They point out the need for more high-quality trials to determine which treatments work.[13]

However, studies did show benefits for:

- exercise therapy
- stretching exercises
- relaxation training
- multi-disciplinary rehabilitation (including physical conditioning, stress and pain management, and ergonomic consultation)
- spinal manipulation combined with massage

In 2000, the Association began an ongoing survey of members about their treatment and its effectiveness.

The results suggest that rest is by far the most effective treatment for RSI, with 90% of respondents finding it effective or very effective. Other treatments that worked well for many people who tried them include:

- stretching
- deep tissue massage
- osteopathy
- walking
- Alexander Technique
- meditation
- Tai Chi
- stress management

Treatments that actually made the condition worse for more than one in five of the people surveyed include:

- swimming
- carpal tunnel surgery
- local anaesthetic injections
- traction (the standout villain!)
- stretches from a physio
- cortisone injections

From the survey, it's obvious that aerobic exercise helps people with RSI. But although both walking and swimming were helpful for many people, more than 20% of people found that swimming actually made their RSI worse.

There are important things we still don't know. For instance, we don't know which treatments work best at which stage of the condition. Anecdotal evidence suggests that rest really only works as a cure early on – when it can be extremely effective. Later on, many people find that rest relieves their condition, but doesn't cure it. By the way, 'rest' means not doing the activities that caused the injury, but otherwise staying active.

We also don't know how to combine treatments to get the best result. But many of our members say that combining an active treatment and a passive treatment – for example walking and massage – works for them.

There's not much in the way of sound scientific explanation for why treatments work. We can speculate that aerobic exercises, such as walking, work by increasing overall circulation to areas of the body – including to the injured area – and that learning healthier and easier ways to use our bodies, such as in Alexander lessons, takes the stress off the injured limbs.

Exercise

We're always being told to exercise more, whether we have RSI or not. We all know exercise is good for you – but many of us don't do much anyway. However, if you have RSI, the extra benefits of exercise make it a vital part of your recovery plan.

When you have RSI, you tend to want to rest your muscles, not use them. That's because using them hurts!

Rest can be very helpful for injured muscles, but even after just a few weeks it can lead to atrophied muscles – muscles that are wasted and weak. That's not going to help you get better.

Most people only think of exercise as a way to lose weight or build up muscle, but for people with RSI, exercise helps to:

- increase strength
- increase energy
- help your body heal faster
- increase self-confidence
- decrease anxiety
- decrease depression

44

- relieve stress
- nourish joints
- keep cartilage, bone and neural pathways healthy

A large body of research now shows that aerobic exercise has strong effects on psychological wellbeing, including depression and anxiety.

Exercise also helps to recondition your body, giving you back the ability to do things you've lost from inactivity. Under-use and inactivity are a real danger when you have RSI – because too much rest has a negative effect on all your muscles, your mood and your circulatory system.

Aerobic Exercise
Aerobic exercise is exercise that works your heart and lungs. It's good for RSI at any stage of the condition. Even early on, when the injury is acute and muscles are constantly sore, going to a gym can be beneficial. Using the exercise equipment (bikes, treadmills and steppers) will improve fitness, mood and, above all, circulation – helping to heal injured tissue faster.

You don't have to go to the gym, though, to get aerobic exercise. There are lots of things you can do, like:

- walking
- swimming
- cycling (exercise bikes are great as you don't have to hold onto the handle-bars)
- running (you may take a while to build up to this one!)
- dancing – e.g. line dancing, belly dancing, Irish dancing
- rollerblading
- sport – soccer, for example
- yoga
- Pilates
- trampolining

- walking in water (good if you have foot or knee problems)
- hydrotherapy: warm water exercise

But I don't feel like it!

We know it's hard to get started. If you're feeling down or depressed, the last thing you may feel like is exercise. But you **will** feel better for it.

> *Exercise gives you a sense of*
> *satisfaction. When you've got an injury,*
> *there are so many things you can't do.*
> *It's good to be able to concentrate on*
> *something you can do. You feel kind of*
> *proud that you've done it.*

It sounds clichéd but one way to get motivated is to stop thinking about it and – just do it! Tell yourself it's only an hour out of your day and you'll feel much better for it (and you will). Allow yourself to achieve something that will make you feel good.

The secret to staying motivated with exercise is to avoid overworking yourself. Exercise at a pace you're comfortable with. You shouldn't feel pain or be completely exhausted afterwards – if you are, try decreasing the distance a little next time. If you haven't exercised for a while, you may find that you're a little sore the next day. This is natural but don't let it put you off. Rest for a day, and then start again.

As your fitness and resistance builds up, you will have to work a little harder. If you start to feel that you haven't exercised at all, then increase the distance or your pace.

Another way to stay motivated is to give yourself a goal that's achievable. You might walk one kilometre three times a week for a month, and then the next month you might walk two kilometres three times a week. It's important to keep your goals realistic. If your goals are too difficult, you won't try. It can help to use a diary system. It's easier to stick to goals if they are written down in front of you – that way you have something solid to work towards. You can also see what you've achieved, and this will keep you motivated.

Other ways to help you stay motivated are to reward yourself, for example with a café stop, make exercise part of your weekly schedule, build variety into your exercise regime and ask friends to join you.

Strengthening Exercises

> *The main thing that helped me was an eight week intensive course which involved lots of stretching and strengthening. As a result of doing this course, I find I have much more mobility than I had before. I would recommend the course to anyone, but I think you have to be prepared to put yourself through some physical discomfort before you see the benefits. It didn't exacerbate my RSI in any way, though there was a lot of muscle soreness.*

Strengthening exercise is often advocated as a treatment for RSI, although the scientific evidence is relatively limited. However, many people do see benefits. "Strengthening exercises, particularly for eccentric strengthening, have been advocated as a treatment for tendon *overuse* conditions since the early 1980s. Clinical studies point to the efficacy of eccentric strengthening regimens."[14]

Strengthening exercise should be combined with aerobic exercise as part of your treatment regime.

However, strengthening exercise is not recommended when:

- you first get RSI (the acute stage)
- your normal daily life is taxing you to the limit

At these times you can still benefit from:

- aerobic exercise
- strengthening exercises for the lower body
- core strength exercises, such as Pilates
- gentle stretches

Taking care of yourself with strengthening exercises

It's essential you don't injure yourself when you start a strengthening program. You need to have an assessment from a qualified instructor or therapist, and you need to be supervised – at least in the early stages of a program. Probably the best type of therapist to help tailor a program for you is an exercise physiologist. This is a relatively new profession, with four years of university training in the field.

Some ideas for making sure you take care of yourself:

- start with no, or very small weights
- talk to your instructor about any pain
- do repetitions slowly and evenly (not in a way that is shaky, fast or inaccurate)
- distinguish between good pain and bad pain (bad pain is pain that lasts, or pain that is not tolerable)
- break up exercises into fewer repetitions (i.e. don't do 30 repetitions in one go: instead, do ten repetitions each time, ten minutes apart, three times)
- use aerobic exercise to warm up before strengthening exercise
- be assertive about what you can and can't do
- give it a try for a fixed period
- try hydrotherapy in warm water

> *When I retired I started playing the piano again – to find that I could really only do it for about ten minutes before I was in pain. Around this time I joined a gym and tried weight lifting, being very careful. After a few weeks, I found that I could sit down and play for 20 to 30*

minutes, which was wonderful.

Choosing a gym

When you're choosing a gym, ask yourself the following questions:

- What knowledge and training do staff have, especially regarding RSI and OOS injuries? They should be able to advise you on the correct technique, which is absolutely vital to recovery.
- Is there adequate supervision? What is the staff-to-client ratio? Are the staff genuinely interested in clients, watching them and checking their technique? Or are they chatting to each other or to clients they like?
- Is all the equipment in good working order, especially bikes, treadmills and other machines?
- Are the air-conditioning and fans too breezy for you? Some people with RSI are very sensitive to air movement on their skin.
- Do they have a good range of weights, especially at the low end of the range? Do they have strap-on weights, for times when you want to minimise strain on your arms? Remember that it's possible to start strengthening exercises by doing exercises without weights.
- What kind of initial and ongoing assessment will you get? How long will the assessment take and how thorough will it be? What are the qualifications of the person who will carry it out?
- How expensive will your program be? Will it suit you better to pay for a complete package, or is it cheaper to come for casual visits?
- Who are the gym's main clientele? Are staff at the gym used to dealing with people with an injury – or are most of the gym's users fitness enthusiasts or body builders? Will you feel comfortable there?
- Is the gym close enough to home or work – allowing you to go when you want to?

Using a gym

When using a gym, remember these points:

- Time other therapies with care around your gym work. Treat anything where you're stretching and strengthening as another gym session. Passive therapies, like massage, are best done soon after a gym session, not just before.
- Remember, as always, you're the one who knows your body best. Tell staff if exercises are too painful or challenging and work with them to find another way.
- When you stretch, you should not feel pain. Stretches should be gentle and held for at least 15 seconds. Stretches are best done at the end of your session.

Talk to staff about the best timing of sessions. It's generally agreed that you need to exercise muscles at least twice a week to strengthen them, and that muscles need a day or two to recover between sessions.

There's some evidence that muscles respond better to strengthening exercises when you consume protein up to an hour afterwards. So eat an egg, some cheese, nuts, meat, yoghurt or a protein drink soon after your session.

Therapies and Therapists

Many people with RSI find that alternative therapies can help to ease pain, reduce muscle tension and promote healing. Most GPs are open to trying alternative therapies and may even be able to recommend practitioners.

Remember that your pain threshold changes throughout the stages of your injury. It may be worthwhile to look at different treatments for each stage. In the beginning, your body may only be able to cope with gentle treatments; later on, however, you may be able to cope with something more challenging.

To help you determine whether or not the therapy is actually working, keep an eye on its effects. Write down how you feel after each treatment and note any changes that occur over the following days.

To find out which treatment is more effective, limit the number of treatments you try at one time. Some people like to limit themselves to one active and one passive therapy at a time. For example, you could try massage (a passive therapy) and hydrotherapy (an active therapy) at the same time.

You should not be in unbearable pain – either during a treatment or afterwards – at any stage of your injury.

Also keep in mind that treatments don't work if you aggravate your injury so be careful about going straight back into the situation that caused the injury in the first place. Speak to the therapist about the best time of day for the treatment, and what work you should do after the appointment.

I have had many positive experiences in the last few years. Mainly I am thankful for all the lovely and caring therapists I have encountered. Their kindness and understanding were invaluable to me, and it has opened my mind to different healing approaches. I come from a very Western medical/scientific outlook with my pharmacy background, but I've now been exposed to a wider range of health approaches, which has done me good. My massage therapist has really held me together, and has been totally reliable and caring – I owe her a lot.

Choosing a Therapist
Choosing a competent, helpful and sympathetic therapist is vital to the success of any treatment. A good therapist will be clear about your treatment plan and the expected

51

outcomes, and help you to feel at ease. Look for someone who:

- empathises with your condition
- is optimistic about the effectiveness of the treatment
- can give clear explanations of what they are doing
- responds to questions and is open to comments from you
- has the appropriate accreditation
- helps you feel comfortable during the appointment

If your insurer is paying for the visits, the therapist may be willing to send the invoices straight to the company.

Questions to ask

Some useful questions to ask a new therapist might be:

1. *Have you treated RSI before? How successful was the treatment?*
   Ask this question when you first contact the therapist. You may like to see someone who specialises in RSI, or has at least had some experience in treating it. Obviously, it isn't worthwhile seeing a therapist who has not been successful in treating RSI.
2. *What exactly do you do?*
   Ask the therapist to explain the procedure and how it will help you. This will give you an idea of what to expect during and after the appointment.
3. *How long will it be before I see results?*
   For most manual therapies, four to eight weeks is a reasonable amount of time to wait before seeing results. Be wary of anyone who tells you that they can fix your injury instantly, or that your recovery will take years of treatment. If the therapy isn't working after a couple of months, it probably won't ever work.
4. *What should I do for myself?*
   There may be exercises or stretches that you'll need to do between treatments. Speak up if the

instructions are unclear or the exercises cause pain.
5. *How should I feel?*
    You generally shouldn't feel a lot of pain after a treatment. However, you might be sore if you've had a vigorous session (such as a deep tissue massage). Find out what a normal reaction would be to the treatment – if it varies too much from what is expected, it may not be the right treatment for you or you can ask the therapist to go more gently at the next session.
6. *How will this treatment work alongside my other treatments?*
    Your therapist should be aware of any other treatments you're undertaking. They may be able to advise you about the correct timing of other treatments, and whether the two will work together.

Evaluating a therapist

If you have followed all the guidelines and the treatment still isn't working, move on to something else. Don't believe a therapist who suggests that it's your fault the treatment is not working – not all treatments work for everyone, and some work best later on when your injury has settled.

Keep in mind that the effectiveness of treatments like massage, physiotherapy and osteopathy can depend on the individual therapist. It may be worth trying a different therapist before giving up completely on a treatment.

And don't stay with a therapist you like, but who is not effective – it's simply a waste of money. As well, keep away from therapists who are flippant about your condition or are not open to your comments.

Try to be open-minded in order to give your therapy the best chance possible for success. If you haven't had any luck with other treatments, you may begin to feel that nothing is going to work. A course in pain management may help by giving you a greater understanding of your pain and how you can live with it better.

Therapies A – Z

Writing about how much is unknown in the treatment of tendinopathies, two Swiss researchers recently wrote "Until now clinical treatment of tendinopathy focuses on physiotherapy (passive or active motion) or anti-inflammatory drugs, e.g. corticosteroid injections (which are largely ineffective and potentially harmful to the patient)… Current therapeutic options for addressing tendon disorders are often ineffective, and the need for improved understanding of tendon physiology is urgent." [15] That's why most people with RSI try many therapies, often finding ones that help but struggling to discover something that cures.

Acupuncture
Acupuncture involves a trained practitioner inserting very fine needles into various parts of the body. They will initially rotate the needles to ensure that they're placed correctly and you should feel a reasonably strong sensation or a very dull ache when the needles are first inserted. However, the procedure will not cause pain. Some people find acupuncture very relaxing. Ask your practitioner about the best timing for your sessions.

The evidence: An international team of experts recently published a report with combined results from 29 randomised controlled trials involving over 17000 patients, looking at the relationship between acupuncture and chronic pain. The results showed that acupuncture is quite effective in reducing pain such as back and neck pain, osteoarthritis, chronic headache and shoulder pain.[16]

The Cochrane Collaboration reviewed acupuncture for fibromyalgia and found nine trials with 395 participants.

54

Some of these trials used electroacupuncture and the rest used manual acupuncture. The authors concluded that there was some evidence that acupuncture improves pain and stiffness in people with fibromyalgia, and that "electroacupuncture is probably better than manual acupuncture for pain and stiffness reduction and improvement of global well-being, sleep and fatigue."[17]

In summary: there is limited evidence for fibromyalgia, good evidence for pain.

Alexander Technique

Alexander Technique is a hands-on postural and movement retraining technique. The sessions will involve guided sitting, standing, walking and sometimes even crawling. You will generally be lying down for half the session as the therapist gently manipulates you. Success depends on the skill of the practitioner, along with your own persistence in carrying out the exercises. The therapist should be able to explain the process clearly and you should see results in a couple of months at the most. A good therapist will teach you how to apply the techniques to everyday life. Alexander therapists can often help you with your office setup, chair adjustment, driving position, and so on.

> *I stopped having massages after nine months because I was relatively pain free. I tried hydrotherapy, but found it an inefficient use of my time – I wanted something I could practice every day. So, I went to Alexander Technique sessions once a week and I believe I improved immediately. It needs constant self-practice to make it work, but it's really worth it. My tolerance levels to vibration and activity increased enormously – as did my ability to do activities that had previously been too painful because of a lower back injury.*

The evidence: There are no large-scale randomised studies regarding the effectiveness of Alexander technique. However, an English study conducted in 2008 observed the effectiveness of combining the Alexander Technique, Exercise and Massage (ATEAM) in over 500 patients with chronic or recurrent pain. Researchers concluded that, when combined, the Alexander Technique and exercise (but not massage) remained effective in reducing pain in the long term, as measured on a disability scale. Number of days with pain and quality of life were also greatly improved among patients participating in this program. The research showed that a short course of Alexander (six one-on-one lessons followed by a supervised exercise program) was almost as effective as having twenty-four one-on-one lessons followed by an exercise program![18]

In summary: there is limited evidence for the Alexander technique.

Bowen Therapy
Bowen therapy is a very light and gentle massage at pressure points that some of our members have found helpful. Sessions normally last 40-45 minutes and you should notice changes in around four weeks. It's an extremely light and non-intrusive therapy that can be helpful if you find normal massage strong or are very sensitive.

Chiropractor
Chiropractors vary quite a bit in their approach, but many use a combination of massage and manipulation.

Cranio-Osteopathy
This is an extremely gentle and non-intrusive form of massage and manipulation that practitioners say encourages the release of tension throughout the body.

Extra-Corporeal Shockwave Therapy
Extra corporeal shockwave therapy (ESWT, sometimes also known as shockwave biosurgery) is a non-invasive method

of treating soft tissue and bone using short, but intense, shockwaves. It's normally done by your GP or a physiotherapist and involves three sessions of treatment scheduled one to two weeks apart. It's normal to feel a 'thumping' sensation post treatment, and you need to avoid anti-inflammatory medications and icepacks for a while. This is because the therapy itself causes swelling in order to stimulate blood flow to the area. You should start to see results at the end of the second week (post-treatment).

The evidence: researchers investigated whether ESWT was effective for rotator cuff injury (in the shoulder). It suggests that ESWT is only effective when used to treat calcific (versus non-calcific) rotator cuff (calcific rotator cuff displays calcium deposits when x-rayed). High strength is most effective in treating calcific rotator cuff (versus low, mid and placebo ESWT), and no improvement was seen in non-calcific rotator cuff cases after ESWT.[19]

In summary: strong evidence for the treatment of calcific rotator-cuff injury using ESWT.

Feldenkrais

Feldenkrais is similar to the Alexander Technique and should be done once a week, for up to an hour. You should see results in about a month. It consists of movement retraining and posture improvement through body awareness. Individual sessions involve some touch and lying down and you will be guided through bodily movements by a therapist. Group sessions, however, involve everyone lying on the floor or sitting and doing guided exercises that increase awareness of movement patterns. This is an intuitive therapy, where you learn by doing each activity. You need to put time aside to practice at home – about half an hour per day. You can expect to move with more ease and less pain if this is successful for you. It can be very effective if you have a good therapist.

Feldenkrais has really helped me with my posture. However, I feel that it needs to be combined with upper body

The evidence: The limited amount of research that is available shows that Feldenkrais can not only be helpful but also very cost-effective with patients suffering from musculoskeletal problems and chronic pain. In one study, 97 industrial workers suffering from neck and shoulder pain were randomly assigned to either physiotherapy, Feldenkrais or no treatment groups for 16 weeks during paid working time. The Feldenkrais group was the only one to show a significant improvement in neck and shoulder pain and in disability during leisure time. The other two groups showed no change (the physiotherapy group) or the complaints worsened (the control group). Two other small studies also showed good results.[20]

In summary: there is limited evidence for the effectiveness of Feldenkrais.

Hydrotherapy

Hydrotherapy is a specially tailored exercise program conducted in warm water under the supervision of a specially-trained physiotherapist. You usually participate once or twice a week for 30-45 minutes. The warm water supports you and promotes circulation, while the exercises help increase strength and flexibility. This is very helpful for sufferers with neck pain and is also useful for building up strength. However, like all strength and endurance training, it can take some months to see results. The exercises are generally not painful at the time, but you may feel tired and a little painful afterwards. While you're exercising, you won't be aware of how hard you're working, so take it easy at first, until you see how you feel afterwards. The pool temperature should be between 33 – 35 degrees so a normal heated public pool is usually too cool.

I found hydrotherapy of great
assistance. Overall, I thought it was

much gentler than physiotherapy
because it put less stress on my body.
Hydrotherapy also taught me about
postural stability and the warm water is
incredibly soothing.

Intra-Muscular Stimulation (IMS)

Intra-muscular stimulation, also known as dry needling, involves the use of a type of acupuncture to stimulate the relaxation and lengthening of shortened muscles, usually carried out by physios. The treatment itself only lasts for a few minutes and it's recommended you receive it once a week.

Unfortunately, there isn't a lot of evidence for IMS yet. One study reported moderate evidence suggesting it was more successful than other treatments for patients with musculoskeletal injuries. However, the study wasn't hopeful that IMS would have long-term benefits in treating the injuries.[21]

"The treatment was sometimes a little
painful. Maarten (the therapist) would
put needles in my back, neck, shoulders,
upper and underarms, and hands. The
impact of each needle could be quite
different: sometimes one or more muscle
contractions, sometimes almost no
feeling was perceived, and sometimes
the effect would radiate to other body
parts. After the treatment I felt as if my
body was in balance – literally as if any
cramps and blockages were removed."
Bas Pronk, RSI Magazine (Newsletter of
the Dutch RSI Association)

The treatment feels different for everyone, and while some report pain from the needles, most people agree that by the end of the process they feel more relaxed and comfortable than before.

Massage

Massage improves circulation, lengthens short and tense muscles and can help to break up scar tissue. We recommend looking for a therapist who has training in remedial or sports massage. It can be quite painful, though a good therapist should be careful to stay within your pain threshold.

Most people like to have a massage once a week initially, then once every couple of weeks when you improve. Your whole upper body will be massaged, but most work will be done on the tightest muscles – probably your back, neck, shoulders and arms. You're likely to have muscle soreness for a few days after a session. If you find that your RSI is worse after a massage, ask the practitioner to go more lightly next time.

Be careful not to overdo activities afterwards. Try taking a warm bath in the evening so that your muscles don't tense up again.

I tried a number of different therapies before a friend in the RSI Association recommended deep tissue massage. At the time I was in a lot of pain, looking after my young daughter, and was completely unable to write. The weekly massage was quite painful at the time, and for a couple of days afterwards, but tremendously beneficial. Within four months I was able to write again and go back to work part-time. I've continued weekly massage since, and have gradually been able to do more and more activities. I feel the choice of therapist is really important, as some are much more effective than others.

The evidence: researchers at a hospital in Madrid separated 100 women with carpal tunnel syndrome into two groups:

the first underwent surgery and the second were treated with manual therapy. The manual therapy treatment involved only thirty minutes a week of massage for three weeks. After a month, the patients receiving manual therapy were actually reporting better results than those who underwent surgery. At later follow-ups, there was no significant difference between the two groups. This implies that massage is just as effective as surgery.[22]

On the other hand, a 2014 Cochrane Collaboration review investigated the effects of deep transverse friction massage for 57 people with lateral elbow or knee tendinitis. The researchers concluded that the evidence for the benefit of massage was inconclusive, though there were minimal reports of adverse effects.[23]

The Ottawa panel, a group of academics which scientifically evaluates physical therapies, found enough data to demonstrate that massage was effective for relieving neck and back pain symptoms in the short term, but there wasn't enough evidence to show any long-term effects.[24]

In summary: there is good evidence for short term benefit, but limited evidence for the long-term effectiveness of massage.

Osteopathy

Osteopaths can vary quite widely in the techniques they use. Some are quite forceful, others very gentle - and some carry out manipulations so tiny you can barely feel them (usually craniosacral osteopaths.) Most osteopaths use a combination of massage and manipulation.

The massage can be fairly deep, which means it may be painful, and the manipulation may be surprisingly forceful. It can include things like 'cracking' your neck to re-align it. While it can be a very helpful therapy for some, if it's carried out insensitively it can exacerbate your condition.

The key is to be as relaxed as possible so the manipulation and massage work to the best effect. Look for an osteopath who is clear about what you can expect. Ideally, massage

61

and manipulation should be given at the same session by the same therapist.

Physiotherapy

Physiotherapists use a range of therapies including ultrasound, traction, manipulation, mobilisation and massage, so what you get at one clinic can be very different to treatment at another. Mobilisation involves the pushing and pulling of joints. Traction is the stretching of the spine manually or by a machine. (Note: machine traction has been known to worsen RSI and is NOT recommended).

Many GPs will initially advise physiotherapy. Some physios see up to eight clients simultaneously – this means that you're actually being treated by the physio for only a short period of time. Some are excellent massage therapists, but find one that will give you some individual attention. A good physiotherapist will not make you do things that increase pain either during or after a treatment. They should explain any exercises clearly and in some detail so you feel confident doing them correctly at home. This is vital because exercises and stretches done the wrong way won't help you.

> *My physio is very hands-on and does quite a bit of massage. She is an excellent teacher and has given me some really useful stretches. Other physios I've seen have mostly used machines, which I haven't found very helpful.*

Stretching

Several studies that looked at workplace stretching programs found that stretching improved flexibility – but only one of these studies focused on injury incidence and severity. The results of this particular study show that people who stretched experienced just as many injuries as people who didn't. But people who stretched regularly experienced injuries which were **less severe**, keeping them out of work for shorter periods of time, compared to people who didn't stretch. Another study showed that stretching combined with strength training gave greater benefits than just strength training alone.

It seems that stretching doesn't prevent injury – at least among the athletes surveyed in research trials. But the jury is still out regarding the question of whether or not stretching helps to **treat** injury.

If you do decide to stretch, the American College of Sports Medicine has recommendations on how to stretch correctly. Firstly, experts agree that you should avoid 'ballistic' stretching – that is, quick bouncy stretches. Hold stretches for around 30 seconds and avoid stretching to the maximum extension. In other words, don't stretch until it hurts, but instead stretch to the point where you begin to feel it, or 'stretch to the edge'.

Secondly, to be helpful, stretching needs to be done regularly, that is, at least two or three days a week. You should repeat each stretch three or four times, and always stretch both sides of the body. The American College of Sports Medicine also recommends being trained and monitored by a professional instructor. We recommend Sharon Butler's book 'Conquering Carpal Tunnel Syndrome and Other Repetitive Strain Injuries: A Self-Care Program' for a very thorough explanation of how to stretch with excellent illustrations.

Swimming

> *At the insistence of my physio, I tried swimming shortly after getting RSI – despite the fact that I had never been very good at swimming. So I got started, in an outdoor 50-metre pool, in the summer. I found coordinating my breathing difficult – and people in the other lanes were, compared to me, swimming to an Olympic standard. I started to feel pressured to swim as fast*

*as I could – which left me feeling
exhausted and disheartened. Swimming
made me sore, not better, and after a
few weeks I gave it up altogether.*

*My second attempt was about eight
months later in a heated, indoor 25-
metre pool. I went during the day, when
most of the people at the swimming pool
were either children or older people –
which made me feel less pressure in
regards to my not-so-good swimming
ability. I took it slow to begin with so I
wouldn't overtire myself, resting at each
end for several minutes before
continuing. I took care to warm-up, and
stopped after only 100m so as not to
overtire myself. I continued this routine
while off work, gradually improving
over 12 months. Swimming became
more enjoyable, and I felt better and
less tight, especially in my neck area.
The key to the success of my second
attempt was relaxing.*

Swimming is often recommended for the treatment of RSI
and overuse injuries, and that's because it's a low-impact
activity which is less likely to put strain on damaged
muscles. Lydia So, a reintegration therapist from the
Netherlands, notes another benefit of swimming: "People
relax more easily in water. Furthermore, you can go at your
own pace."

Majon van Eijsden, a specialist in rehabilitation, says that
for swimming to be successful in helping with RSI, posture
is very important. "Most people bend their head too far back
in relation to their torso, especially with freestyle or
breaststroke." Van Eijsden advises that people swim on
their backs because, if it's done smoothly, this is a less
taxing stroke.

Taking it easy is easier said than done. When I was first advised to take up swimming, I could hardly swim at all. When you are in constant pain, you tend to avoid movement – and chronic inflammation of my shoulder made it impossible for me to move my arms. Despite this, I persevered – using a neck-float so that I only had to use my legs. Initially I tried to swim at my old pace – I really suffered after that first time. So I would advise anyone to be satisfied with three laps at first. Intentionally swim in a relaxed and slow manner, and be creative – don't dismiss a therapy or activity if it does not work out immediately, but find a way to make it work for you

You may feel pain in your muscles after swimming, especially if you haven't exercised in a while, but the pain should fade fast.

Van Eijsden comments:

"If it hurts, you have to slow down and modify your action. I always give my patients the following rule of thumb: within two hours' time the pain should be back to its basic level. If this doesn't occur you've gone beyond your limits – and you should do less next time."

Remember that training needs to be built up very gradually, even if you're not suffering from pain. If you don't take it easy, swimming may worsen your condition.

Ideas from our members
- Normal swimming uses mostly upper-body muscles. Try using flippers to take some strain off your upper body.

- Switch between strokes, to evenly exercise all muscles and avoid putting strain on your neck. Try overarm, side-stroke, breast and backstroke, and walking in the water.
- Rest between laps if you're tired
- Goggles and a snorkel help to keep your neck comfortable
- Be careful not to crane your neck back when doing breast-stroke and freestyle.
- Try walking in water – it's good exercise and the pressure of the water helps to open your chest.
- Your muscles relax much better in warm water – see if you can find a well-heated pool.
- Begin with a warm-up, such as walking up and down the pool, and end with a soak in the spa or a hot shower to relax your muscles afterwards.
- Try doing most of the work with your legs and just moving your arms through the motions *without* pulling.
- Opening your fingers also helps to reduce the strain on your arms.

> *Wearing a snorkel means I don't have to turn my head to breathe. This means I'm not struggling to turn my head and I'm not squashing my shoulder and neck muscles to get my head around. My swimming action is smoother and longer – my head isn't bent, I can breathe and I suffer less pain. As for swimming on my back, I find that my neck gets extremely tired and painful – so I'm now trialling a neck-rest that floats.*

If you aren't comfortable with swimming, or if even these precautions we've talked about make you sore, try something less strenuous. Other exercises such as simple walking or hydrotherapy may be more appropriate for you, as each person's injury responds individually to different forms of exercise.

Most importantly, remember that if swimming makes you sore for more than two hours – or if it's stressful or tiring in any way – slow down, change your action and do less next time! Remember to think of any exercise you do as rehabilitation, not fitness training – so only do as much as you're comfortable with.

Injections for RSI

There are a number of treatments for RSI that involve injections of one substance or another, some experimental, like platelet-rich plasma, others well-established, like cortisone. In this section, we look at the evidence for each of these treatments.

Platelet-rich plasma (PRP) or 'blood spinning' has been around for over 20 years. Initially, the treatment was used to speed up recovery from some types of surgery, usually dental or facial reconstruction procedures. About ten years ago, doctors started using the therapy as an alternative to more invasive surgery or drugs to treat stubborn sports injuries that weren't responding to traditional treatment. These days, the procedure is most often used to treat overuse injuries or tears in tendons around the knee and other joints.

The idea behind PRP is that platelets are the body's natural healing tools because they contain growth hormones which help body tissue to regenerate. In the procedure, blood is removed from the body, spun in a centrifuge and reduced to a high-concentration platelet solution. It's then re-injected into the body to act as a catalyst in the healing process.

The effectiveness of the treatment is largely undocumented and subject to debate, with the vast majority of positive results being purely anecdotal. A recent double-blind study in the Netherlands, published in the Journal of the American Medical Association, investigated its use in the treatment of chronic knee problems. In this rigorous study, some patients were given PRP and others received an injection of a saline solution, with researchers finding no significant difference in pain levels after two years.

67

The evidence: A Cochrane Collaboration systematic review covered a number of clinical conditions including rotator cuff tears, shoulder impingement syndrome, elbow epicondylitis and a range of tendinopathies. They concluded that "there is currently insufficient evidence to support the use of PRP for treating musculoskeletal soft tissue injuries".[25]

Another systematic review looked at the medical literature on the efficacy of platelet-rich plasma injections for tendinopathy at the elbow and found "strong evidence that PRP injections are not efficacious in chronic lateral epicondylar tendinopathy".[26] [27]

In summary: so far there is no evidence for the effectiveness of PRP.

Hyaluronic acid (HA) is a naturally-produced compound in our bodies found in muscular tissue, skin and cartilage. It has many roles within the body, including being the main component in synovial fluid (a substance that reduces friction between cartilage in certain joints). It's also an important part of articular cartilage and a major component of skin, where it's involved in tissue repair. A 70kg person has, on average, about 15 grams of hyaluronic acid in their body. As you age, hyaluronic acid production decreases and this is thought to be a cause of skin ageing and increasing joint pain as we get older.

HA has become a common additive in cosmetics that claim to reduce the signs of ageing. The USA Food and Drug Administration first approved it as a cosmetic filler in 2003, and since then many other products with hyaluronic acid have been approved as well. It's thought to work by helping skin absorb water more efficiently.

In 2010, Canadian researchers studied the effect of hyaluronic acid on people with tennis elbow. After studying over 300 patients, the researchers found that the group treated with HA achieved significant improvements in grip and return to normal function. There was a high degree of both patient and physician satisfaction with the treatment.

The Canadian researchers were very pleased with the results, reporting that the treatment had great potential due to its low risk and the rapid recovery of the patients who were treated. [28]

The side effects of HA are minimal, with very few patients reporting any adverse effects. For injections, common short-term side effects include bruising, swelling, pain and tenderness at the injection site.

From our reading, HA from creams is not well absorbed into the body and is unlikely to be of any use in tendinopathy. Unfortunately, it seems you really do need an injection.

Cortisone injections looked like a miracle treatment for overuse injuries in the late 1940s when the drug was first synthesised. They're extremely effective for quickly relieving the pain of tennis elbow, carpal tunnel syndrome and shoulder injuries and are much used in the treatment of sports injury, but even early clinical trials raised doubts about how effective they were in the long term. A recent article in the Lancet has confirmed those doubts by looking at over 40 trials of cortisone injections, mainly for rotator cuff (shoulder injury) and tennis elbow.

All of these were good quality studies which compared thousands of people who received a cortisone shot with others with the same injury who were either not treated or followed different treatments. It turns out that cortisone is effective for fast pain relief that may last weeks, but when patients are followed up six or twelve months afterwards, it's a different story. Their chance of a relapse was 63% higher than people who received no treatment, and they had a much lower rate of complete recovery.

People who had more than one injection had even worse results. "An average of four injections resulted in a 57% worse outcome when compared to one injection," according to the lead author, Dr Bill Vicenzino of the University of Queensland.

In a commentary accompanying the article, Dr Karim Khan from the University of British Columbia said that the use of cortisone is a result of a misunderstanding of the fundamental nature of overuse injuries. He points out that the evidence for exercise therapy "is more encouraging than the evidence for corticosteroid injection." Dr Vicenzino commented that sodium hyaluronate "demonstrated vastly superior results across all time points" and he believes it's worth further study.

In summary: no evidence for the effectiveness of cortisone injections in the long term.

Medicare Savings

If you have a chronic condition, there are quite a few ways to save money through Medicare.

'Gap' Costs

Firstly, it's important to be aware that once you have paid a certain amount of out-of-pocket costs (the exact amount depends on your Centrelink status), Medicare will cover 80% of the out-of-pocket costs for all medical services provided *out of hospital* in each calendar year. You should register for this initiative by visiting your local Medicare office. It's important to register ASAP, to make sure that all of your gap costs are included. Expenses incurred before the date of registration are not included in this benefit. Gap or out-of-pocket costs include, for example, the difference between what you pay your doctor and what you receive back from Medicare.

Saving on Medicines

If you spend over a certain amount on PBS medicine (prescription drugs covered by the government-subsidised Pharmaceutical Benefits Scheme) within one calendar year, you can get the rest of the year's medication at a cheaper rate, or for free. However, the amount you need to spend equates to about one prescription a week, so many people will not qualify. If you're a Medicare card holder, and you and your family spend more than $1317.10 on PBS drugs in a calendar year, your subsequent PBS medications will cost $4.70 each. Concession card holders (with a Centrelink or DVA concession card) and their families paying $4.70 per script can get free PBS medicine once they've spent over $336.00.

What to do

- Ask your pharmacist for a Prescription Record Form (PRF), on which they record each PBS medication purchase.
- Once you've reached the threshold, ask your pharmacist for a Safety Net card to get your discounted or free PBS medicine.

Make sure that you...

- ensure that information is recorded correctly
- tell your pharmacist once the threshold has been reached
- store the card safely

Things to watch for

- pharmacists can charge a 'recording fee' of over a dollar each time.
- if you get the more expensive brand of the drug, rather than the generic, the difference in cost isn't covered by the Safety Net. To avoid this, ask your doctor not to tick the 'brand substitution not permitted' box on your prescription.

Medicare Rebate for Psychologists' Fees

The Medicare rebate has recently been extended to private psychologists' fees, making it much more affordable to be treated for anxiety, depression and other mental health disorders. The system is very similar to what happens when you see a GP – the rebate covers 85% of the schedule fee. However, psychologists - like doctors - sometimes charge about 40% higher than the schedule fee. So you can still be paying something out-of-pocket, and while this is difficult for some, it's an improvement. You can claim on *either* your private health cover or through Medicare – not both – and for most people, this new Medicare rebate will far exceed their private rebate. The Medicare rebate can be claimed on up to 11 sessions a year. If you're a Health Care Card holder, the cap on 'the gap' limit will apply – in other words, after you reach this threshold you will no longer have to pay anything for sessions in that year.

Saving on Allied Health

One of Medicare's best-kept secrets is that limited benefits are now payable for services from eligible allied health professionals. Information about this scheme is difficult to obtain and many GPs are not keen on the paperwork involved so we hope the following summary will assist you.

Eligibility: You're eligible if you have one or more chronic conditions.

Benefits: A partial rebate may be received for up to five services a year from allied health professionals if these services are provided under a General Practitioner Management Plan (GPMP). If you have significant dental problems related to your chronic condition, you can claim up to three services a year for dental care. For other services, you cannot claim more than five services per year – beginning from the date of the first service that you claim under the scheme. If you have private health insurance, you can claim a benefit under your private health fund *or* Medicare, but not both.

Allied health professionals include: physiotherapists, chiropractors, osteopaths and psychologists, audiologists, chiropodists, dieticians, mental health workers, occupational therapists, podiatrists, speech pathologists, dental practitioners, dental specialists and Aboriginal health workers. These professionals must be registered with the Health Insurance Commission (HIC).

For more information, ask your GP, your local Medicare office or contact the Department of Health and Ageing on 1800 020 103.

CHAPTER 4
PAIN - WHAT YOU CAN DO

Simple Ways to Reduce Pain

Firstly, if an activity causes hours of pain, find another way to do it or just stop – but remember to keep moving to maintain circulation and promote healing. Then modify your activities to reduce pain. A log of activities, postures and pain can be useful in targeting activities that are a problem, such as hanging clothes on the line.

Cold

Cold can be very effective in reducing inflammation and pain and is best used immediately after the activity that triggered pain. Cold running water can help to ease pain, or you can apply ice directly to the affected area in short intervals of 40 to 60 seconds, with no more than 10 to 15 applications of ice per day.

Don't let ice sit on your body – make sure you move it along. Apply it to muscle and avoid bony areas, such as the point of the elbow. After you have used cold water or ice, let that area of your body heat up again slowly and naturally before you start an activity again. About 10 to 15 minutes would be the right amount of time.

Heat

Heat can be a great way to relieve pain. This can be applied in various ways, including heat packs, heat-wheat packs, warm water and hot water bottles. You can use a hot bath or shower to relax sore muscles.

A long hot bath can help to set you up for a good night's sleep, and a hot shower can help to start the day in less pain.

TENS

Transcutaneous electrical nerve stimulation (TENS) can be helpful, especially if your pain interferes badly with your capacity to sleep. It involves fitting pads to your body which stimulate nerves electrically – this stimulation interferes with pain signal transmission. You can hire a TENS machine from a pharmacist.

Massage

Massage by a physiotherapist or masseur is a very effective way of relaxing muscles and reducing pain and has been very effective for many people with overuse injuries. If you find regular massage too painful, Bowen Therapy is very light and may be helpful.

Self-massage is another simple form of pain relief. One way of massaging your arms is to roll a hard rubber squash ball between your arm and a table; the ball can also be used to massage your back and shoulders against a wall. Battery-operated massagers are another option.

Medications

Medications can play a useful part in managing pain. However, it's generally not a good idea to use painkillers to enable you to continue doing the activity that is causing your injury; this masks the pain signals your body sends to let you know that damage is occurring. Remember that all medications have some side effects, especially if used for a prolonged period. Along with this, some people have low tolerances for certain medications. It's a good idea to visit your doctor regularly so they can keep an eye on how you're going with your medication.

Psychological and multidisciplinary approaches to chronic pain management are other options to explore. Many major hospitals run useful and helpful free pain clinics that are very effective. As well, some psychologists have particular expertise in pain management, working with you to find useful strategies.

If pain is interfering with your sleep, seek medical help. Overall, pain management is a skill you learn over time.

Creams, Rubs and Herbs

Most of us have tried one cream or another to relieve the pain we get from our repetitive strain injury. But what's in these creams? Do they have side effects? Most of the commonly available creams and rubs fall into four categories:

- those that contain non-steroidal anti-inflammatories
- those that contain salicylates (a substance closely related to aspirin)
- those that contain capsaicin
- counter-irritants

Whether **non-steroidal anti-inflammatories** are effective for pain resulting from overuse injury is controversial. However, if you want to take anti-inflammatories, and are concerned about their side effects, the dose is lower in creams and this will reduce side effects. You may be able to avoid stomach and gut problems by using a cream on your skin as opposed to taking anti-inflammatories orally. However, it's important not to use a cream and a pill together – your risk of side effects would be much higher. You shouldn't use anti-inflammatories at all if you're pregnant or breastfeeding, have kidney problems, asthma, stomach ulcers or digestive problems. These creams include Diclac, Difflam, Feldene Gel, Orudis and Voltaren Emulgel.

It's thought that **creams that contain salicylates** work in much the same way that aspirin does to decrease inflammation and relieve pain. Don't use them if you're allergic to aspirin or are on blood-thinning drugs. These creams include: Deep Heat Arthritis and Night Strength, Dencorub, Linsal, Metsal, AR Heat Rub Cream and Liniment ARF.

Some creams and rubs contain capsaicin, a substance that occurs naturally in chillies. Unlike most of the other creams and rubs, there's actually some scientific evidence to back up their effectiveness. Capsicain contains a substance that interferes with the pain signalling system, and it's been shown to be effective in helping relieve pain from osteoarthritis. It's worth giving these creams a try over a period of time, as capsaicin becomes **more** effective the more you use it. When you start using it, it can cause a burning sensation, but this tends to disappear as you continue. Products include Zostrix and Finalgon.

Counter-irritants are thought to work by producing a sensation that diverts your attention away from the pain. Not a very convincing explanation, but these creams certainly work for many people. Some products warm the skin and others cool it. They're generally considered pretty safe, even for pregnant or breastfeeding mothers. Products include Tiger Balm Red and Goanna Heat Cream.

> *I find Tiger Balm, both Red and White, very effective for pain in my neck and shoulders. It seems to relax the muscles and relieve the pain. Once or twice I made the mistake of putting it on straight after a bath, and this was much too hot!*

All of the above creams and rubs can cause side effects, including allergic reactions on the skin. Which one you choose will depend on practical considerations and how effective they might be for you. For example, some of them are quite smelly, which can actually be a good way of letting other people know that you're not feeling great today. Others can stain your clothing, while some claim to be non-staining. Some lose their effectiveness over time and that's when it's a good idea to try another one.

Herbal Remedies for Pain and Healing

While lots of people use 'natural' remedies, there hasn't been a lot of research done into their effectiveness. This situation is changing, however, with the National Health and Medical Research Council recently committing millions of dollars to researching these remedies. Also, in Germany, a government-appointed body called Commission E produces reports on the effectiveness of traditional remedies.

A report in *Choice* magazine looked at herbal plant-based remedies that claim to promote wound healing or reduce pain, including arnica, calendula, tea-tree oil, papaya and lavender oil, all of which have a long history of use.[29]

Evidence regarding the effectiveness of these remedies is patchy but encouraging nonetheless:

- **Arnica**, as a herbal (not a homeopathic) product, has been shown to be effective for osteoarthritic pain by increasing blood circulation and reducing swelling.
- **Calendula** has been shown to accelerate healing and is thought to reduce inflammation.
- **Tea tree oil** has been shown to reduce inflammation in some small-scale studies.
- There's not a lot of good quality research regarding the use of **papaya**, but there is some evidence that it has anti-inflammatory properties and relieves joint and muscle pain.

All of these plant-based products can cause allergic reactions and skin irritation but otherwise seem to be very safe.

If You Have Chronic Pain

Approaches to chronic pain have changed a lot over the last few years in response to new scientific evidence on the body's responses to injury. These new conceptualisations of pain look at the effects of pain on the nervous system, in which pain messages are interpreted as danger signals. When pain becomes chronic, danger signals are continually pumped into the body, and the operation of the nervous system is fundamentally changed. Chronic pain therefore "rewires" the nervous system.

> *"To me, being a pain psychologist for quite a few years already, this particular model has really filled in some missing pieces of the puzzle, and its doing so for my own clients as well."*

This gives rise to a new approach in managing chronic pain. Just as *pain* can "rewire" the nervous system, *you* can succeed in "rewiring" your nervous system to better manage pain. This new approach is based around three practical interventions you can take to start "rewiring" your nervous system and thus learn to manage your pain more effectively. These are **movement**, **relaxation** and **pacing**.

Chronic pain is partly a dysfunction of the immune system. The role of the immune system is to immobilise the body when injured, sick or in danger. For example, when a person has the flu, they become more sensitive to pain, their mood deteriorates and they experience stiffness, fatigue and changes in temperature. This is an immune response to the flu. The immune system has immobilised the body to aid healing and allow it to safely increase the body's temperature to deal with the virus.

Similarly, after an acute injury, the body responds with pain, lower mood, stiffness and fatigue. There may also be slight changes in temperature. We tend to immobilise the injured body part. This is an appropriate and helpful response to a short-term injury. However, we also tend to respond in a similar way when an injury becomes chronic.

Are You Immobilising When You Don't Need To?

People with chronic pain often stop moving the areas that are giving them pain and may not be aware they are doing so. They think movement is painful, therefore dangerous, and the painful part of the body needs to be immobilized. For acute pain, immobilisation is necessary, but for chronic pain, it's not.

> *"If you have chronic and constant pain, observe how you move to see if you're not already immobilising parts of your body. It can be very subtle."*

The first practical intervention is to start moving

This new approach to chronic pain employs feedback loops to start "rewiring" the body to better deal with pain. For people with chronic pain, the feedback loop is simple. You immobilise because you're in pain, but immobilisation, in turn, tells your body you're in pain. This is an automatic immunological response. You need to consciously and deliberately "rewire" the body to reduce your suffering.

Movement is key to the functioning of our nervous system. While stretches and exercises are good, you need to start moving in a conscious and deliberate way, to start "rewiring" the nervous system. *"Nerves that fire together, wire together"*. Once nerves fire together in a particular direction, they keep firing together in that direction.

> *"For someone like me with 20 years of lower back pain, my pain experience has changed completely since I've started using these techniques."*

You need to do two things when it comes to movement. You need to:

✓ **Normalise movement**
Immobilisation rarely relieves chronic pain, and we believe, in fact, that immobilisation actually contributes to pain. If you move normally, this

demonstrates to the body that pain is unnecessary and you will start to "rewire" your body and your nervous system.

✓ **Increase movement**
While too much movement will cause pain, too little movement will also do the same. When you start moving, do not move too much or too little. You need to activate the nervous system in an adaptive way: try gently wiggling and jiggling where it's painful.

> *"I remind myself that my back is there, my back is moving and that it's okay. I actually say out loud to myself, "Yep, my back is here, my back is moving, and it's okay". In as many ways as you can, you need to start "rewiring" your body."*

The second practical intervention is to relax.
The danger reaction is the natural "fight or flight" reaction when a person is facing imminent danger. This is the sympathetic nervous response: adrenaline kicks in, breathing goes to the upper chest, blood flows out to the extremities, the digestive system stops working, heart rate increases. This is great for immediate danger, but not so good if it goes on for a long time.

The body is always trying to achieve homeostasis, or balance. Following a sympathetic nervous response (the danger response), the nervous system then activates the parasympathetic response (the relaxation response) and relaxes the body, and fatigue follows,

This is the body's way of restoring balance. For people with chronic pain, however, their nervous system is continually bombarded with danger signals, stimulating a constant sympathetic nervous response. They do not experience the usual parasympathetic response that follows.

"I've conditioned myself. So I just have to say the word, "relax, breathe", and I get really sleepy."

Learn to relax. The nervous system needs to be "rewired" back into experiencing the parasympathetic response. Relaxation techniques are essential here. Fear of movement is a conditioned response that you need to override. You can start to pair movement with a relaxation response instead. If you can trigger the nervous system to relax when you have pain, then you remove the danger message and avoid going into the full-blown immune response.

Breathing is key. There are other relaxation methods but learning to relax through breathing is a simple and easy technique to start practicing. The aim is to practice breathing until you can think "breathe" and you relax. When we breathe in, we activate the sympathetic system, and when we breathe out, we activate the parasympathetic system. When facing imminent danger, breathing goes to the upper chest, taking long breaths in and short breaths out. A person in pain will often breathe like this.

You need to train your breathing to do the opposite. Breathe in for a count of one, and out for a count of two. You will activate the sympathetic system slightly, but the parasympathetic system more, and you will relax. You need to practice this technique all the time, not just when you're desperate, but when you have little or no pain at all. Practice until you can employ this technique automatically and calm your system.

How do you know when to stop when you're in pain?

For people with chronic pain, certain activities will often cause pain. For these people, pain becomes their "stop" signal. Sometimes pain can be delayed so a person will often stop "just in case" the next time around. For people with chronic pain, pain is saying "stop" *all* the time. Generally, a person with chronic pain will always check their pain before undertaking an activity. They are thus restricted by an operating system which is pain-driven.

For people who don't have chronic pain, "go" is normal. There is no need to check for pain. Pain has a function in this basic operating system, because it signals a person to stop if they are injured to allow time for their injury to heal. In general, however, for these people, pain is not the main factor. Their basic operating system is based on **choice.** They choose when to stop, often after a certain distance, time or repetitions. For example, at the gym, a person may decide to do 20 pushups, and even though it may start to hurt after 5 push ups, they don't have to stop. They can make a choice to push on through.

But for a person in chronic pain, this system doesn't work. They have lost their choice, and instead, their decisions are driven by pain. If you have chronic pain, you rely on pain to know when it's safe to move or not. So to get back to a normal way of operating, you need to "rewire" your nervous system, remove pain from the equation and return to a system based on choice.

> *"It took me about 2 years to shift my nervous system and immune response. Now it works to my liking. It doesn't mean that I don't have pain. It doesn't mean that I don't get flare-ups. But my pain flare-ups have gone from 3 weeks of immobilisation to 3 or 4 days with full movement."*

The third practical intervention is to start pacing.

You need to start with time and use an accurate stopwatch.

- Select an activity. Choose as many as you want, because the more you train, the more you **can** train and the more effective pacing is. For example, you might choose walking.
- You will have a baseline of pain. Start your activity and note the time when the pain starts or increases, not when it becomes overwhelming. For example,

after 10 minutes of walking your pain begins to increase.

- Take a number of readings and then take the average. Reduce this time by 30%. You have effectively taken pain out of the equation. With this 30% buffer, you can do the activity with confidence and by choice. For example, you walk for 7 minutes with confidence and then you stop by choice.
- Continue to practice the activity with your 30% buffer until you're bored with that timeframe.
- Increase the timeframe by 10% and practice again until you're bored. Continue to increase by 10%.

"Rewiring" the nervous system is a long process, but if you stay with the program then your baseline of pain will eventually increase. But don't be overconfident when increasing the time frame. You can also work with repetition and distance, but always plan ahead and be careful.

> *"Chronic pain is like the dark side of neuroplasticity, but what I'm saying is this is the bright side of neuroplasticity, this is how we can rewire ourselves to live a better life. Chronic pain has already rewired your nervous system so you are going to have to retrain it back."*

Practice, Practice, Practice.

Practice is key. You need to practise normalising and increasing your **movement**. You need to practice your **relaxation** techniques. You need to practise your **pacing** activities. When you practise these three practical interventions, you're successfully "rewiring" your nervous system to better manage your pain and achieve a better quality of life.

Our thanks go to Randolph Sparks, clinical psychologist, for his help with this section.

Coping with Flare-ups

A flare-up can hit you when you least expect it. For the last little while, you've been able to manage at work reasonably well and you can do a bit more at home too. You've even started to feel that maybe you're on top of this RSI thing and you might recover. And then, with no warning, the pain hits you again! It's depressing and frightening. You think "Am I right back where I began? What am I going to do?"

You're not alone. Everyone with a pain condition has flare-ups. They do happen, and they're hard to cope with. However, they are manageable.

The first thing is to work out whether it's an aggravation or a flare-up. Answering 'yes' to the following questions might indicate an aggravation:

- Do you have symptoms in a new area?
- Do you have new symptoms?
- Are your symptoms out of control?

If it's an aggravation, then you will need to visit your doctor and work out what is going on. You may need to really pull back on activities in order to give your body a chance to recover. Ask your doctor about new therapies you can try during this time to reduce aggravating your symptoms.

Deciding that it's a flare-up can be pretty discouraging too. You may start to feel anxious and panicky because life has suddenly become unpredictable again.

However, there are things you can do. First, work out what caused the flare-up:

- Have you been doing more than you should – taking a 'crash through or crash' approach?
- Have you been more stressed than usual?
- Have people been pushing you to do too much?
- Have you been too conscientious or too hard on yourself?

- Is there a new tool or activity in your life, or have you been doing something in a different way?

A useful way to narrow down the cause of your flare-up can be to keep a pain diary (see Chapter 3 for more details).

Of course, it may just not be possible to work out what caused the flare-up at this stage. In that case, keep it as an open question at the back of your mind and an answer will most likely come to you.

Once you've worked out the cause, then you know what to change and you can develop a plan of action. You plan should include strategies to both physically and emotionally manage your flare-ups.

For some people, a flare-up will cause panic, while others prefer to ignore it in the hope that it will all be okay. Generally, neither of these approaches works. Instead, you need to see your flare-up as a problem you can solve. That is, you need to change your approach from 'panic' mode or 'it will all turn out alright eventually' into 'investigating and finding solutions' mode.

Physical Solutions

Sometimes we can get back on the road to recovery (or at least the road to well-being) by just changing what we do. Pacing, varying and cutting back on activities – especially those that are most painful – can be the solution.

You should also think about your current treatments. Some of them may be making your injury worse during a flare-up. You might need to modify treatments like stretching and strengthening until you start to feel better. This could be a good time to treat yourself to a massage.

> *"I frequently get flare-ups across my shoulders. The things that help me manage the pain include doing small shoulder movements as much as possible to loosen them up, using heat packs and paying for a massage. If they*

don't work, then I use a strong painkiller
as a last resort."

You can also use strategies like using heat or cold (whatever works for you) to dampen down pain. Other things that can help include Epsom salts in a long hot bath to relax your muscles or a brisk walk to keep up your spirits.

Emotional Solutions

When we are in pain, we often don't want to talk about it, and withdraw from the people around us. Taking some time out might work for some of us, but for many, it's better to stay in touch with the people who make us feel good and care about us. Instead of spending a lot of time talking about how depressing it is to be in pain again, plan to do something enjoyable together, like seeing a movie, going for a walk or watching your favourite sport.

If you feel you need counselling or help with pain management, you may be able to get a referral to a specialist psychologist under Medicare from your doctor.

Relaxation

Learning to relax can be a very helpful way of coping with pain. Yoga classes often teach this, but you can also download some really good relaxation scripts from the web. For example, you can find a helpful script from the ABC here:
www.traumacenter.org/resources/pdf_files/relaxation_exerc ises.pdf

Another useful technique for both relaxation and chronic pain management is practicing mindfulness. Mindfulness is a popular psychological technique which teaches you to become consciously aware of your thoughts, feelings, sensations and behaviour without being weighed down by them.

Your doctor can refer you to a psychologist who specialises in teaching this technique for those with chronic pain, or

87

you can try a mindfulness class. You can also download some excellent mindfulness scripts from the web.

If you start feeling panicky, there's a technique called '5-4-3-2-1' that some people find very helpful.

The aim is to 'ground' yourself by stopping, slowing, naming and noticing. Just take a break and notice:

- Five things you can see
- Four things you can hear
- Three things you can feel, like your feet on the ground and your hands on your lap
- Two things you can smell (or would like to)
- Then take one long slow breath

Focusing on your breathing is another quick and useful technique to help yourself calm and relax. Focus on slowing your breathing and lengthening your outbreaths. As we've said, there is a scientific basis behind this: when you breathe out slowly, your parasympathetic nervous system kicks in. The parasympathetic nervous system (nicknamed the 'rest and digest' system) functions to relax and slow the body down. It does this by decreasing your heart rate and reducing muscle tension so you don't notice as many physical signs of panic or pain.

Communication

You may need to change the way you communicate to cope well with a flare-up. This could be a good time to practice asking for help. Are you too independent to ask for help from people who in fact would be very willing to give it? Do you feel shy about asking for help?

At work

If the cause of your flare-up is connected with work, you may need to think about changing how you communicate. For example, do you need to learn to say no? Or maybe allow yourself to ask for help? Do you need to get better at prioritising work tasks?

In practice, these skills can be hard to learn and difficult to try out. You could try talking over and practicing these strategies with friends or with a professional counsellor or psychologist.

Be careful!

In order to cope with the sadness that a flare-up can make us feel, it's common to reach out for that extra glass of wine, box of chocolates or packet of chips – whatever comfort food is available. Don't go overboard on these – they're only a short-term fix, if that.

Avoid making any big decisions while you're feeling bad, and put off any discussions that could be stressful. You won't be at your best and it can be hard to think clearly and stay calm.

Applying these Ideas

When you're in pain it can be hard to step back and develop a plan of action. So, you can (mentally) prepare a pain flare-up toolkit. This could be just a list on the fridge that reminds you about the things you can do that will help the condition, improve your mood and help to distract you from the pain. Some suggestions include:

- people who cheer you up
- DVDs of your favourite comedies
- an MP3 or CD player with some guided relaxation or mindfulness scripts
- some bath salts for a long relaxing bath,
- heat packs or heat rubs
- pain medication (if you use this too often, it won't be as effective when you really need it – like during your flare-ups!)
- a pleasant place outdoors to walk or sit
- some money set aside for a massage, sauna or spa
- our self-massage links
- books that make you feel good

- easy recipes or frozen meals

Remember that your flare-up is only temporary and that it will pass.

And finally…

Try to learn from your flare-ups so that you can prevent them from happening again

CHAPTER 5
STRATEGIES

*They were funny little things like I
couldn't manage chopsticks and I
couldn't roll spaghetti with a normal-
sized fork because it was too heavy. I
couldn't keep my hand up in the air to
hold it.*

*Even now, I have to stand back and
think about changes that can be made.
For example, I recently asked myself –
does my baby still need to use the high
chair? I decided that she was ready to
use the kid's table and chairs I'd bought
– which means that I don't have to lift
her into the high chair. I look at each
activity and ask myself, 'is this the best
way?' If I decide it's not, I find or invent
another way.*

Learning New Ways to do Old Tasks

One of the major impacts of RSI is on your capacity to
perform the ordinary tasks of everyday life – things like
cutting vegetables, opening doors, turning taps, hanging
washing on a clothesline and even dressing yourself can
become very difficult. It can also be hard to come to terms
with not being a fully independent adult.

Trying to learn new ways to perform old tasks can be very
frustrating. It will help if you have support – moral support

91

from others who suffer from RSI and have learnt to adapt their approach to everyday tasks, along with practical support from family members who recognise that they need to do more, and professional support from a counsellor to help you through this difficult period.

Many other people with RSI have had to meet these same learning challenges so there's a fair bit of knowledge out there already. The experience of others can be a good resource for you, helping you to find ways of simplifying your own life.

The following strategies give you ideas for some changes you can make in your daily activities, but you can find many more for yourself by reading and talking with other people who have RSI.

Tackling Difficult Tasks

There are four broad ways of looking at tasks that you find difficult.

> Don't do it at all
> Get someone else to do it
> Change the way you do it
> Use special equipment.

It's a good idea to make a list of tasks you find particularly difficult. Look at each task and ask yourself these three questions:

- Does it really need to be done? If not, don't do it. If yes, then prioritise the task.
- Am I the best person to do it? Re-allocate, share, roster, exchange tasks.
- What is the best place and time for this task to be done?

Getting Organised

- Set up things to reduce the strain (e.g. in the kitchen, store frequently-used items closer, and rarely-used items further away).
- Move tasks to the warmer part of the house.
- Have double sets of items to avoid carrying (e.g. cleaning supplies kept in both the kitchen and the bathroom).
- Only put the quantity you need into containers like the kettle.

In *The Arthritis Helpbook*, the authors outline a method of problem-solving that helps many people with arthritis.[30] Their suggestions are just as relevant to people with RSI so we've included an adapted extract here. There are eight steps, as outlined below.

Step 1. Identify what is difficult for you.

Think about the last 24 hours. Which tasks were problematic for you? If this is hard to pinpoint mentally, try writing down everything that you've done. Tick the things that were difficult, painful or made you feel tired.

Step 2. Pinpoint the reason for the problem.

- What part of the task made you sore, tired or stiff?
- How fast did you do the task? For how long were you able to do the task?
- Why couldn't you do it as well as you'd have liked? Is pain the reason? Not enough movement? Stiff? Not strong enough? Worried about what others would think?

Step 3. List ideas that might help. Ask your family and friends for ideas.

Step 4. Choose an idea you think will work. Try it.

Step 5. Check how you went. Did you solve the problem completely? If you still have problems, try the next step.

Step 6. Try other ideas from your list. Check how you go each time. Keep going until you run out of ideas.

Step 7. Find out more. Get some more ideas from the RSI Association, therapists or books.

Step 8. Accept that you might not solve the problem now. The problem-solving you have already done might be helpful later.

An Example of Problem Solving...

Identify	I can't open jars.
Problem	Sometimes it's painful; I'm too weak.
List Options	Ask spouse or neighbour.
	Buy cans and use an electric opener.
	Buy a jar opener.
	Use a sheet of rubber to produce more friction by placing over the lid.
	Run the lid under the hot tap.
	Release suction with a knife.
	Tap strongly with a knife around the lid and then open it.
Choose	Tried to release suction.
Check	Worked on some jars but not others.
Choose	Buy a jar opener.
Check	It's wonderful!

Pacing and Switching

*A big plus for me with this whole
episode has been my change in attitude
towards work and my lifestyle in
general. I have learnt to respect and
listen to my body. I take life a lot more
slowly, and I certainly don't take my
health for granted anymore.*

*I used to think that the only way to get
things done was to do everything at once
so it was a hard lesson to learn to slow
down and to learn to focus when I had
to put things down and pick them up
again. I had to curtail my impatience.
But I was finally learning to work with
my RSI and becoming more efficient.*

Budget your energy!

Many books on RSI talk about 'budgeting' the use of your
upper body. This means conserving your energy and not
over-working muscles. While this sounds reasonable, it can
be difficult to achieve. Before RSI, you were able to
complete tasks as you wanted or needed. But you now have
to find new ways of working that won't aggravate your
injury. This can be difficult and frustrating.

How many times have you completed a task and been in so
much pain that you couldn't do anything else for the rest of
the day, or even the rest of the week? More often than you'd
like to think? It's easy to work yourself to that point. You
still want to work at the pace you were working before RSI,
but you can't. Instead of limiting yourself to what you can
do, you push yourself and aggravate your RSI.

This scenario probably sounds familiar to you. However, it
doesn't have to be this way – there is actually a system that
limits pain and aggravation, called *pacing and switching*.
This process can be applied to all situations that are

repetitive or likely to cause you pain. It's very simple and easy to apply.

Pacing and switching requires you to break down tasks into small, manageable parts. These parts are interspersed with rest or other tasks that use different muscle groups. By pacing out tasks and switching between them, you're less likely to aggravate your injury.

The hardest part of dealing with RSI can be admitting that you have an injury – and working with it, rather than working *against* it. Pacing and switching are techniques that help you to work **with** your RSI. They give you the ability to take more control of your injury by combining work with rest.

Pace yourself
Pacing means breaking up a task into parts and resting between each part. By pacing, you're not completing a task in one block. Instead, you break it up into parts and rest between each one. This way you're staying within your pain threshold and not pushing yourself too far. An important part of this process is stopping any task *before* you feel pain. Once you feel pain, you have gone too far. At this point, it's unlikely you will be able to do anything else until it subsides.

However, it's often difficult to know when you have overworked yourself. Many people with RSI don't feel pain until later in the day, or even the next day.

One way to overcome this problem is working to the *70% rule*. That is, do 70% of what you *are* capable of, not what you *think you should* be capable of. Then, stop and rest to conserve your energy and prevent pain. If you apply the 70% rule, you will be stopping a task before you put yourself at risk. Therefore you should never work yourself to the point of pain. Essentially this rule gives you control over your pain levels.

Switching

Switching means changing between different tasks so that you don't tire out one group of muscles. You complete one task using a certain muscle group and then switch to another using a different muscle group. This requires you to be aware of your body and which muscles are used for different tasks.

Here are a couple of examples of how this works:

1. Instead of trying to clean the whole bathroom at once, you could break it down into four parts – shower, bath, floor and basin. In between each part (or even halfway through each part) stop and rest, preferably for at least five minutes (this will vary depending on your needs). Depending on the extent of your injury, you may want to do two parts one day and two parts the next day.
2. At work, you could break tasks down into small parts and mix them up. You could type a letter, then make a phone call, then do some stretches, then do some filing. Each of these jobs uses a different set of muscles.

This technique can be applied to any situation. The rules are the same for any task that is repetitive or is likely to cause you pain – break it down into manageable pieces and do one piece at a time.

Pacing and switching sound simple; in reality, they can take a while to get used to. It may mean changing your priorities and your standards. For example, you may not be able to get the whole house clean in an afternoon. But remember, the most important thing is being well.

If having a spotless house means you're in pain for a week, is it really worth it? If you clean the house over a couple of days or even a week, you're conserving energy to do other things that you'll enjoy more.

You will also have to experiment with the process. This is where a pain diary can help. It can be helpful to write down all the tasks you want to get completed. Then, add sleep time, rest time and socialising. This will help you to see exactly what you want to do and figure out how achievable your plan is.

There is no point in being in pain if you don't have to be, so don't push yourself too hard. Working harder doesn't mean you get more done, especially when you have RSI. Take lots of short rests and allow your muscles to recuperate before commencing the next task, or continuing with the previous one.

> *I learnt the miracle of pacing. The more breaks you take, the more efficient you become. You need to let go of the desire to have everything completed right away.*

You need to work *with* your RSI rather than *against* it. Using pacing and switching helps you to work more efficiently. This means that you have taken a step towards managing your RSI.

Some tips for pacing and switching

- Set out what you want to get done at the beginning of the day or week. Be flexible – recognise things may not get done and that's OK!
- Break jobs down into manageable bits. If possible, list them so you can refer back.
- As you do each task, remember to pace and switch. Be conscious of how much you have done and what you're capable of.
- Having lots of small rests is more effective for conserving energy.
- Stop any task before you feel pain.
- If you do feel pain, stop immediately and rest.
- Work to the 70% rule, that is, do 70% of what you're capable of doing (not what you think you should be doing) then rest or switch.
- Note how you're feeling after each task and write this down.

- Think about what is more important to you – pushing yourself to get something finished or being able to enjoy your day without pain.
- You may need to experiment with the process at first but remember to stick with it – over time, you will become more aware of exactly when you need to rest or switch.

Day-to-day Living

This section deals with issues such as driving, writing and reading, as well as a number of other tasks that we all need to do on a daily basis.

Reading

Reading is an everyday task that can be painful with RSI but there are ways to make it easier. The first thing to remember when you read is to maintain a good posture. Craning your neck over to read makes your muscles work hard to support the weight of your head; this can also compress nerves to the hand and arm.

One way to bring the level of the book closer without using your hands is to mount the book on cushions or a 'stable-table' on your lap. This also makes it easier to tilt the book towards you, rather than bending your neck over. If you're reading at a desk, a tilt board (the same as you would use for writing) does the same thing.

One member says, "Be cruel to books! Depending on the type of binding, they can be difficult to hold open. Bend them back until the spine snaps and they'll yield more easily."

Here are a few more handy tips:

- hardbacks are generally easier to hold open than paperbacks
- lying books open face-down, and then piling more books on top is a good way of loosening the binding

- library books or used books from second-hand stores are generally already well-worn, which makes them easier to hold open
- There are a few gadgets around that take some of the work out of reading, such as a high-backed reading chairs with proper neck support and a page-turning device that straps onto your arm with an extension to help you turn the pages. The rubber end of a lead pencil can be dragged across the page if pages are difficult to separate. A rubber thimble does this too.
- A page-holder to hold pages open while you read; we recommend the "Gimble". A book-stand holds the pages open and tilts the book at an adjustable angle – recipe book holders are cheap and hold books at a good angle. A recommended bookstand is the *Brilliant Book-rest.*

Driving

Driving can cause pain in the arms, neck and shoulders. But you can change things in your car to make driving easier and safer for you. Firstly, it's important to be as relaxed as you possibly can.

If you're buying a car, think about these features:

- power steering or rear-wheel drive to make steering easier
- automatic transmission so your hands are both free for steering
- a good match between your body, the controls and seat. You need to be able to control the vehicle while in as comfortable a position as possible. Some people find it helps to sit quite close to the steering wheel (check requirements for your air bag)
- a "smart key" system – this will allow you to open the car and start it without actually inserting your key into the lock; it's great for people who have difficulty with keys

- a dash-mounted gear change – much easier to operate than a floor-mounted system
- a rear-view camera for reversing
- a foot-operated parking brake.

The ease of power steering and central locking varies between models. So try before you buy – take the car for a test drive and open the boot, doors and petrol tank to test how much effort is required.

Of course, buying a new car with all the extras is not always a realistic solution. Some more affordable adjustments you can make to your existing car include:

- steering wheel covers that make the wheel much easier to grip, especially ones that make the wheel substantially thicker, like lambswool covers
- key-holders to make car keys easier to handle
- wide-angle mirrors, like the ones used when pulling a campervan, increase the amount of rear vision and reduce the need to crane your head around
- some RSI sufferers find the pull of the seatbelt on their shoulder uncomfortable. You can use a lambswool seatbelt cover to relieve the pressure and warm the upper shoulder

Apart from adjusting the car, you can adjust the way you drive. Some of our members' driving habits include:

- driving through to the opposite parking spot so you don't have to reverse out
- using two hands to pull up the handbrake
- making sure you're as relaxed as possible when driving
- checking that your shoulders are loose and that you're holding the wheel gently
- varying your hand position often
- ensuring that you have proper lumbar support for your back

As with all of the activities that have been covered here, if it causes you pain then the best thing to do is avoid it. There's always public transport, which has the added benefits of being economical and environmentally friendly.

Please also remember that you must feel safe and confident with the driving style you adopt. **If you don't feel that you have full control of the car, don't drive.**

Public Transport
Public transport can also cause some problems, particularly at peak times. If you do have to stand up on a bus or train, try the following:

- loop your arm around the pole instead of holding onto it with your hands
- place your bag between your feet, rather than trying to hold it.

Opening Doors
- Push doors using your hip, shoulder or feet
- Pull a door open by standing close to the door, turning the handle and walking backwards – holding your arm still
- Revolving doors should be moved by pressing on the outer edge where there is more leverage, or letting someone else go first
- No doorbell? Tap with your umbrella or something similar, or lightly tap the door with your foot. Alternatively, call on your mobile phone to let the person know you've arrived
- Elevator buttons can be pushed with an elbow or knuckle
- Keys can be covered with a keyholder to make them easier to grip and use
- At home, invest in special handles to cover the doorknob, and spray *Ezi-Glide* onto stiff locks and knobs to help them turn more easily.

Carrying
- If you use a shoulder bag, carry it across your body

- Look for backpacks that put weight on the hip (they have a band at waist level)
- Don't carry unnecessary items in your bag
- Look for big pockets in parkas, vests or jackets
- Buy a pair of cargo pants and use the pockets to carry keys, wallets, etc.
- Use firm containers like baskets or boxes which can be carried close to your body and rest on your hip or stomach
- Waist packs are available from outdoor shops
- Bumbags are useful and you can find ones that are very small and neat
- Use trolleys (e.g. laundry trolleys). You can take small parcels of wet clothes to the laundry basket outside.

Watching TV
Be careful how you sit when you're watching television. Make sure you have a good chair with lots of support so that you don't have to crane your neck or back.

Shaking Hands
Shaking hands with another person can cause a lot of pain. But avoiding a handshake just feels rude!

- don't worsen your condition just to be sociable
- say something like "sorry, sore hand!"
- try coming up with a new idea that doesn't hurt your arms, e.g. touch forefingers
- shake hands very loosely

Clapping
Applauding is another task that can cause pain. Try these instead:

- lightly tap your palm with a program
- whistle, or shout 'Bravo'
- mime the action instead of actually doing it
- stamp your feet

Travelling

Some hints to help you with travelling are:

- Plan ahead – for example, remember to pack warm clothes if cold aggravates your overuse injury.
- Stay at least two nights in each place; this will limit packing and unpacking and generally make your stay less rushed.
- Identify where you want to stay, the activities you want to do, your methods of transport and the assistance you need. Choices range from a fully-catered cruise, where you get off at each destination to go sightseeing (minimum effort meals, activities, housekeeping, transport and childcare) to backpacker-style hostel and coach travel trips (self-sufficient meal purchase, preparation, activities, bed-making, repeated packing and unpacking, and luggage handling) or even camping.
- Schedule extra time for yourself so that you can rest and take a break.
- Pack your heaviest items closest to the wheels of your suitcase. This makes the suitcase more stable and easier to pull.
- Leave lots of time to make transfers, move your luggage, and stretch and move around.
- Travel light. Consider mailing some of your luggage or purchases home.
- Take quick-drying clothes that you can hand wash and drip-dry.
- In advance of your trip, let the plane and train carriers know that you need assistance.
- Pack lots of small bags, one with just your overnight needs, for car travel.
- Pay extra for linen & towel hire.

Using the Phone

- Headsets are the easiest to use.
- Cordless models stop you cradling the phone, and you can change your position regularly.
- Try using the speaker.

- Look for a phone with light touch keypads or use a pencil to operate an ordinary phone.
- Use your phone's memory to minimize dialling.
- Get a hands-free set for your mobile. That way you can put the mobile in a bag or pocket and still talk.

You may be able to get free or discounted equipment through your telephone company's disabilities service.

Sleep and RSI

Sleep problems affect many people in today's society - in fact, a recent study found that 12% of Australians experience chronic daytime sleepiness. As many as 32% of people experience insomnia or sleep disturbances and this figure is even higher among people with a chronic illness.

Tiredness

Researchers believe that tiredness is a growing problem in the modern world. In 1911, the average night's sleep was 70 minutes longer than today! Of course, not everyone *needs* the same amount of sleep. Although 8 hours is a rough guide, if you find yourself needing 9 you're not unusual. Also, women, on average, need an hour **more** sleep a night than men.

You can tell if you're not getting enough deep sleep because you'll feel tired through the day, have poor concentration levels and experience more aches and pains. This is certainly not helpful for people with a chronic injury because they have enough pain as it is. Sleep also promotes healing and reduces stress levels. So let's now look at isolating possible *causes* of low sleep levels because poor quality sleep can be caused by a wide range of factors.

First of all, it's important to deal with things that impact negatively on sleep such as alcohol, cigarettes and caffeine. Nicotine is a stimulant so if you're a smoker, taper off during the day. Although alcohol can help you drop off to sleep, it actually lowers the quality of your sleep and messes up your sleep cycles. This means you don't end up getting enough deep sleep - the true remedy for continual tiredness and fatigue. Finally, caffeine in any form is best avoided after 4pm. Switch to decaf drinks in the mid-afternoon to get to sleep. Blue light from screens can also make it hard to get to sleep, so get your computing done earlier in the evening.

RSI-affected people certainly know that pain doesn't help when bedtime comes. During the day, exercise and activity often help people cope with chronic pain. The daytime is generally a busy time anyway so there are plenty of things to help divert your attention away from the pain. At night, however, pain may come to the foreground and make it hard to sleep. Heat can be really helpful in relieving local pain. An over-the-counter pain-relieving medication may also help. A pharmacist suggests that pain relievers work best if taken *when the pain starts*, not when it becomes overwhelming. Another way of relieving pain at night is to use a TENS machine (try one out before buying if you can–they don't work for everyone). Talk to your GP for advice on night-time pain management.

Let's now look at the widely promoted remedies for poor sleep, including sleeping pills. While taking them may seem like a good idea, sleeping pills can be addictive. In fact, Beyond Blue recommends that you don't take sleeping pills for more than a week for this reason. Next up are the natural remedies, particularly herbal remedies like valerian. These may work for you, but you shouldn't use these for an extended period of time (i.e. when you have chronic insomnia). Remember to tell your GP if you're taking any natural remedies because they are still medicinal products.

Sleep experts recommend what's called 'sleep hygiene' and it works for many people.

The basic principles of good sleep hygiene
1. Have a regular rising time and a regular bed time. This is one of the **most** important ways to improve

sleep quality. People with sleep problems tend to develop the habit of sleeping in or napping to 'make up' for lost sleep. But every time you sleep in, you give your body clock a tiny dose of jetlag that takes 3 days to recover from! Your body actually compensates naturally for under-sleeping one night, by making you sleep more soundly the next. It's a good idea to keep your sleeping hours the same every day and never sleep in by more than half an hour (even on weekends!). So if you have a late night or trouble sleeping, it's best to put up with feeling a bit tired the next day and keep your body clock finely tuned.

2. Avoid eating for three hours before sleep – but eat before that so you don't go to bed on an empty stomach!

3. Try not to do anything stimulating for at least 30 minutes before going to bed, Save that un-put-downable thriller or tense discussion for the following day.

4. If you can't get to sleep, try not to force yourself to sleep.

5. After about 20 minutes, if you find you still can't sleep, get up from bed and find someplace comfy to sit – maybe in front of the TV or perhaps with a good book. The bed should only be used for sleep and sex so that your body knows that the bed is for sleeping in (and not tossing and turning in). Try to do a calming activity until you feel sleepy again. Then return to bed, and repeat this cycle if you wake up again.

6. For people with chronic pain, make sure your bed covers are light and don't weigh down on painful joints or muscle areas.

7. Try not to let stress about daily things interfere at bedtime because there is absolutely nothing you can do about any issue at night other than to worry about it pointlessly. The daytime is a more practical time for problem-solving. One good way to deal

with night-time worries is to write down everything that worries you before you go to bed.

8. Try to make your bedroom quiet, dark and cool and avoid overdoing the blankets—excess heat can stop you from getting 'deep sleep'.

9. You'll sleep better if your body temperature drops as you go to sleep. So a hot bath an hour before bed and keeping the bedroom cool can both be helpful.

Stress, depression and sleep problems

Stress is certainly no friend of sleep, and you may find yourself losing sleep when you're stressed or going through a hard time. It's important to note that lack of sleep can also be a symptom of depression or anxiety. Visit www.crufad.org or www.beyondblue.org.au to learn more about depression and anxiety and see your GP to obtain a referral to a qualified psychologist. *Beyond Blue* also has several good fact sheets about depression and sleep, which you can access directly from them, or from us at the Association.

Pillows

I have always slept on cheap polyester pillows until recently, and I'd noticed increasing neck stiffness. On my partner's recommendation, I bought a memory foam pillow that is sculpted to fit the neck and designed for sleeping on the side. It's a very heavy pillow and cost $85 but was certainly worth it! I'm sleeping much better and my neck hasn't given me any trouble since. I also find the pillow to be perfectly comfortable if I sleep on my back.

For people with an overuse injury, being able to sleep well and wake up without pain is important, and having a comfortable pillow can really help. The right pillows depends partly on your sleeping position. Stomach sleepers should try a low, soft pillow while if you sleep on your back, a medium-to-firm pillow might suit you. If you sleep on your side, you will need a higher firm pillow.

Generally, your pillow should support your head so that your spine is in a straight line - and this means a pillow that's not too low or soft, but also not too high or hard.

Many of our members find that a pillow with a depression for the head and support for the neck is very helpful in preventing neck pain. Some find that sleeping with the chin closer to the chest seems to help prevent neck pain.

I place a cervical roll (a long foam cylinder), 52 cm long and 5 cm in diameter inside the pillow case along the edge with a regular pillow. I find that this extra neck support makes a big difference to how well I sleep. It's easy to take on holiday too. (Cervical rolls are available from McKenzie Products on +64-4-299-7020.)

I have tried many pillows, most of these continued to cause me neck pain, along with very strong headaches and migraines. The biggest problem when finding a pillow is that you generally can't return a pillow to the store if you don't like it - which means that finding a pillow can be a very expensive exercise. I recently found a pillow which I would thoroughly recommend to any person who suffers from RSI and neck pain, called a 'Chiroflow Waterbase Pillow'. It contains a water pouch underneath a layer of polyester fibre. The real advantage of this pillow is that the water pouch means that its height is adjustable, unlike any other pillow. It is also supportive but very soft, which is perfect for sufferers of neck pain. It only took me a week of using this pillow for my neck pain to dramatically decrease.

Housework

- Your employer's insurance may cover both house and garden help.
- Hire help or barter for help. If you can't afford a weekly cleaner, employ someone to do the hard work once a fortnight or even once a month.
- Build up the grips on houseware, e.g. by wrapping towelling or bubble wrap around the handle on mops, brooms, and other tools.
- Do small parts of the work throughout the week, for example and clean one room at a time so that you limit your time on each activity.
- Have carpet removed (hard floors are easier to clean).
- Move your body as a whole to decrease pressure on your arms. For example, when sweeping the floor, walk the broom with your whole body rather than just pushing with your arms.

Making beds

- Buy a two-sided duvet cover so you can turn it over instead of washing it.
- Use a piece of board with a handle (such as a table-tennis bat) to tuck in sheets and blankets.

In the laundry

- Wash small loads often.
- A front-loading washing machine doesn't tangle clothes and creases them less. It will also get them drier. Some machines have very high (1300rpm) spin cycles, which means washed clothes are drier and lighter to carry.

- Hang clothes as soon as you can after washing, to reduce creasing.
- When ironing, iron only the areas people can see, such as the front of shirts.
- Use a lightweight iron (e.g. a travel iron available from travel shops).

Hanging washing
- Try to swap new spring pegs with old ones from your friends or try dolly pegs - much easier to use!
- Hang or peg the garments on hangers, and then lift them up onto the line. When the clothes are dry, you can hang them in the cupboard without folding or ironing.
- If it's not windy, just hang clothes over the line without pegs.
- Dry your clothes on a clotheshorse or plastic clip line.
- Use a laundry trolley to get clothes to the line.

In the Kitchen

Labour-saving foods
- ready-grated or sliced cheese
- pre-chopped tomatoes (in cans and cartons)
- pre-chopped ginger, garlic, lemon grass, chilli and herbs
- ready-made sauces
- pre-chopped vegetables from the supermarket
- frozen sliced or chopped onion
- frozen pastry
- ready-made pizza bases
- pre-sliced or diced meat
- frozen vegetables or vegetables that require little preparation e.g. Brussel sprouts, baby squash, baby carrots, snow peas, cauliflower, broccoli
- sliced bread

Carrying food
- Carry things with both hands where possible.
- Use your open palms to lift and carry.
- Slide cookware along benches on a tea towel.
- A kitchen trolley is very useful for gathering things and taking them to where they will be used.

Avoid carrying whenever possible. A laundry trolley can also be used to carry groceries from the car to the house and to take garbage out to the bin. Remind yourself that it's always better to make two trips rather than overloading yourself on one and paying the price.

If you don't have someone to help you with shopping, you may be able to use a telephone ordering and delivery service, or shop online. Alternatively, it's better to do the shopping several times a week as opposed to just going once a week because then you only have to carry and lift smaller amounts. Choose a supermarket trolley that runs properly and use it to transfer shopping to your car.

Storing and easy access
- Keep drawers running smoothly by rubbing them with candle wax or by spraying with a little *Ezi-Glide*.
- A Lazy Susan can be useful in cupboards or on the bench.
- Baskets or shelves fitted to the inside of the cupboard doors provide more accessible storage.
- Pack shelves in accordance with use - nearer to waist level for things you use the most.

Keep frequently used items on the benchtop. You can buy a storage rack that will keep all your crockery neatly on the bench in a small space. Storage racks can create extra space in cupboards.

Pouring liquids
- When pouring liquids or draining vegetables, stand the kettle, jug or saucepan on the edge of the sink on a non-slip mat or wet dishcloth - then, place the

container in the sink and pour. In this way, you can tip the kettle or saucepan without having to hold its weight.

- Use smaller, lighter jugs and teapots.
- Put only as much as you need in containers.

Making tea and coffee

- When making tea or coffee for yourself, just heat one cup of water in the microwave.
- Fill your kettle or electric jug using a lighter plastic jug.
- Put a hose attachment on the tap for filling the kettle.
- To make taps easier to turn, have them fitted with special washers designed for people with arthritis.
- Use a tea bag squeezer to remove the tea bag from your cup – it requires only a light, easy grasp.
- Carry the teapot or kettle on a trolley or a tray.
- Choose a lightweight kettle which is easy to pour from or try a kettle or teapot tipper.
- Use a lightweight glass or cup that can be grasped easily.

Knives

Use the 'power grip' whenever possible - this means making your hand into a fist so that the handle of a utensil rests against your palm. Small implements you would normally hold with just your fingers and thumb can be very painful to use. However, if you cover the handles of these with firm foam padding, you can hold these using the power grip.

The Power Grip

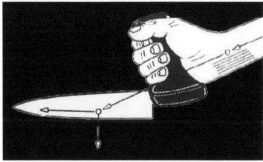

The *Stirex U-knife* is specifically designed for people with hand or arm problems. It has a large and comfortable easy-to-grip handle at a 70° angle to the blade.

For cutting foods like steak, it's essential to use a very sharp knife and a serrated blade can also help. Store your knives in a knife rack rather than in a drawer as it will keep them sharper for longer. There are always electric knives, too.

Opening cans

An electric can-opener can help here, but try before you buy.

Ring-pull cans can be opened by applying leverage with a spoon or with a special ring-pull opener.

Opening jars and bottles

There are various approaches you can take to opening jars and bottles. Some of these include putting the lid under hot water before trying to open it, purchasing a special jar or bottle-opening tool, or using a thin rubber mat to grip the lid. You can stabilise a jar (or can) for opening by putting it in an open drawer, and leaning against the drawer.

Use one of the following types of jar and bottle openers:

- Those which work to improve hand grip on the lid - a piece of sandpaper or non-slip matting can be used for this job.
- Those which operate on the leverage principle.

- Under-shelf mounted jar openers. You need to be sure you have a convenient place to put this. Do not position it above chest level. You can hold the jar with two hands for this method.

Opening milk cartons and packages
- Cut the top off the milk carton using a bread knife or scissors and pour the milk into a jug. When pouring, hold the jug with both hands.
- Use a knife to cut a cross in foil-topped cream or yoghurt containers, and then peel back the corners.
- For liquids in cartons, you might try a carton spout. These punch an opening in a milk carton and provide a pouring outlet.

Washing up and wiping up
- Let dirty dishes soak first or use a dishwasher if you have one. Ideally, a dishwasher should be installed about 50 cm from the floor to make loading and unloading easier.
- Buy extra-absorbent cloths and use both hands when wiping.
- If liquid spills on the floor, drop a towel and use your feet to wipe up.
- Dry the bottom of your cups by placing a tea towel over all the cups in your dishwasher when draining.
- Use newspaper on benches to catch spills.

Preparing meat, vegetables and fruit
- Don't peel anything unless it absolutely needs to be peeled.
- To peel an onion easily, pour boiling water over it and leave for ten minutes, drain, and the skin will slip off easily. The onion can then be chopped or sliced in a food processor.
- For pumpkin, try part-cooking it in the microwave before peeling or cutting it.
- Buy washed potatoes - small ones for boiling in their skins and large ones to bake in their jackets in the oven or cook in the microwave.

- Include the family in cooking–it can be lots of fun for little ones to get involved.
- Cook in foil to cut washing up.
- Each time you cook, make a larger amount so that leftovers can be frozen and used later.
- Your food processor will chop up just about any vegetable into small pieces. It will grate soft vegetables, like zucchini, and will mash up tomatoes. If you want to process something soft or sticky, put it in your processor with something harder. For example, if you're using herbs in a recipe, you can chop them up with the onions quite successfully - likewise, raisins can be chopped with nuts. If you decide to buy a food processor, make sure it's easy to turn on and off, doesn't require continuous pressure to stay on and is easy to disassemble and clean. If it moves around on the bench, use a rubber mat underneath.
- Use kitchen scissors to cut up herbs and sliced meat like bacon.
- Buy a lightweight peeler with a wide grip. When you're peeling, try to incorporate short breaks. Also, try to have several different types of peeler handy in the kitchen so you can use each one alternately for the same job – this helps give your hands a break.
- You can use foam rubber or buy some cheap tubing to build up the handle of kitchen utensils – such as cutlery and peelers – to help make them easier to use. The *Goodgrips* range of utensils have large, soft handles that make holding easier.

Stirring
- Use the power grip when stirring food during cooking. This is where your wrist is straight and you grip with your whole hand. It's the easiest grip for someone with RSI.
- A balloon whisk with a wide handle can be particularly useful for stirring. For turning food

during cooking, try self-opening turner tongs - these tongs only require a gentle grasp to close them.

- Have a non-slip mat, a damp dishcloth, or a soap grip handy. These can be used under bowls and saucepans to help stabilise them.
- Try working with the bowl or pan at a lower height, such as in the sink.
- Use a mixing wand with an on/off button that does not need to be pressed continuously.

Draining vegies, rice and pasta

- Use a steamer or steamer insert in a saucepan to cook vegetables, or use a microwave oven. This means that you only need to cook in a small amount of water, and you won't need to lift heavy saucepans.
- Take cooked vegetables out of the saucepan with a slotted spoon.

Making cakes, biscuits and pastries

- To make cooking things like pies and tarts easier, try using frozen pastry. Not only is it kinder to your hands, but it's also practically 100% failure-proof!
- Use lightweight cookware.
- Use mixing bowls with pouring lips and handles.

For guests

- Forget about trying to impress guests, and lower your standards to a level that suits what you can manage – and still have a good time yourself!
- Order a plate of sandwiches from your local deli or bakery.
- Ask your guests to help with carrying, setting the table, cooking at the BBQ, etc.
- Eat outside to minimise cleaning up.
- Make the occasion as informal as possible.
- Go out to eat, invite friends back for wine and cheese or dessert.
- Use paper or plastic plates.
- Stick to simple dishes when you're entertaining.

117

- Accept any offers of a food contribution!
- Use a no-iron tablecloth or placemats.

Looking after Yourself - Personal Care

Hygiene
- Soap dispensers in public facilities are often empty and waste hand energy. Instead of bothering with these, carry disposable hand wipes.
- Using an electric toothbrush may help, but be aware that some models vibrate much more than others. Look for a good thick handle.
- You can buy a pump dispenser for toothpaste; this may be easier than squeezing a tube.
- Invest in good-quality nail clippers, or try using punch clippers.

Clothes
- Buy skirts and pants with elastic waists.
- Dress in layers so you don't have to manage heavy garments.
- Use knee-high stockings, or buy devices to help put on socks and pantyhose.
- Avoid zippers and troublesome buttons - you can buy button fasteners in specialty catalogues. Alternatively, you can use a coat hanger or hook to pull your zip up.
- Instead of laces, buy slip-on shoes, or shoes with Velcro or elastic fastenings.
- Try stretch laces for shoes.
- Knit fabrics are easy to wash and put on, and they often don't need ironing.
- Hang your clothes up after each wear to reduce the need for ironing.
- Using a tumble-drier also reduces the need for ironing.

Hair Care

- Unscrew the top of the shampoo bottle so you don't have to squeeze it.
- When you're brushing or blow-drying your hair, hang your head down and don't raise your arms.
- Support your arm on a table when you're brushing or drying your hair.
- Use a wide-tooth comb for dealing with knots and tidying your hair.
- Cut your hair shorter.
- Buy a hair towel; these absorb more water than normal towels.

Your sex life

Sex can be difficult with RSI, and many people find that they have a lowered sex drive. However, RSI certainly doesn't have to spell the end of your sex life.

One of our members suggests that sex can be helpful in managing RSI – despite the fact that when you're in pain sometimes you don't even want to be touched. Taking the first step towards having sex (or even being more intimate) can help you to overcome some of the depression associated with RSI.

Here are some pointers to keep your sex life going:

- Make sure the room is warm – don't restrict yourself to the bedroom if another room is warmer.
- Communicate with your partner; he/she needs to know what you can and can't do.
- Be creative and experimental - you may not be able to use the positions you used before so come up with some new ones which don't require you to place any pressure on your arms.
- Find other ways to please each other - buy a book for tips and advice, there are lots of great resources out there!
- Sit up for foreplay (and sex), this way you maintain better circulation in your hands and arms.
- Use your mouth and lips instead of your hands.

- During sex or sleeping, don't lie in a position which cuts off the blood circulation to your arms or hands.
- Try letting your natural desires and feelings take over for a while rather than concentrating on your RSI.

If you haven't had sex for a while, you could try working your way up to it slowly as follows:

- Try just touching each other's bodies - concentrating on relaxation.
- Even if it's too much to massage your partner, ask him/her to massage you – concentrating on relaxation at first and then moving on to more sexual feelings when you're ready.
- Continue to build on your feelings until you're comfortable enough to take it to the next step. It can take time for you to feel comfortable enough to have sex again, so be patient.

Using a Computer

I got RSI when computers, and the idea of doing your own typing, were being introduced to the department. Although I could type, I wasn't sitting in an ergonomic position, and my chair did not provide adequate support. Alongside this, I was given a laptop as my personal computer. When the end of financial year came around, I was working at a fast pace, as well as taking work home at night and studying using the laptop. It got to the stage where I couldn't type more than a few minutes at a time and couldn't keep up with the workload.

Typing is not a natural position to be in. I am a big guy and it's hard to be

Keyboarding

Firstly, keep your hands in a straight line with your arms – don't curve them in or out. Keyboard trays and split desks limit your options, so they're not a good idea.

Alternative keyboards have been designed to minimise the hazards of computer use but not all of these work well. The negative slope keyboard has the potential to increase wrist extension and to keep users in one fixed position. However, it's increasingly recommended by ergonomists as a way of reducing RSI.

Split keyboards, for example the **Kinesis** keyboard, help a lot of RSI sufferers but they do take a while to get used to! In general, ergonomic keyboards give better results if users like using them.

Is the right angle really right?

In the standard poster on the 'correct way to sit at a computer', the calves are at a right angle to the thighs, the thighs at a right angle to the trunk, the forearms at a right angle to the upper arms. But is this really the best way for a human being to sit and work at the computer? These days, many experts say no.

For example, a very high quality study was carried out in 2002 which, despite its age, has much to offer computer users. The researchers followed 632 newly-hired computer users who were just starting work in eight large organisations in Atlanta, USA. None of them had any prior musculoskeletal symptoms and all of them anticipated using a computer for at least 15 hours a week. Over that year, more than half of the participants developed upper body musculoskeletal symptoms related to their work.

During the study, the researchers collected data on participants' posture and computer setup, while participants themselves kept a diary on how many hours they used a computer each week, other hand-intensive activities and their symptoms. In this way, it was possible to work out which postures and ways of using the computer led to musculoskeletal symptoms.

Neck and shoulder symptoms

To avoid pain in this area, elbow position was important – participants whose elbows were below the keyboard were more likely to suffer from musculoskeletal symptoms of the neck and shoulders. The ideal angle at the elbows was more than 120°, with arms sloping downwards to the keyboard. Twisting the shoulder out more than 25° to reach the mouse was also associated with increased symptoms. Using chairs with armrests was associated with fewer symptoms, while using a shoulder telephone rest caused more problems.

Hand and arm symptoms

Here, the position of the keyboard was crucial. People whose keyboards were higher were at greater risk, as were those whose keyboards were closer to the edge of the table. Having the "J" key on the keyboard more than 12 cm from the table edge was related to fewer symptoms. Using more force on the keys was associated with an increased risk of disorders, as was turning the wrist inwards to use the mouse. Surprisingly, using a keyboard wrist rest was a definite risk factor. Monitor height made a difference, with fewer symptoms for those whose heads tilted downwards to look at the monitor.

The authors conclude "in the light of the results of the current study, the seated position traditionally recommended for computer users – upper arms perpendicular to the floor, elbows kept at a right angle, forearms parallel to the floor and the keyboard at or above elbow height and near the edge of the disk tray – may not be the lowest risk posture. Although promulgation of this posture is widespread, it appears to have gained its near universal acceptance without epidemiological evidence of its efficacy."

What about the traditional advice to sit with your back at 90° to the chair seat? According to Cornell University ergonomics web, this kind of erect sitting is "NOT relaxed or sustainable". They recommend a posture where your back is at an angle of 100 to 110° from vertical. This is when "the chair starts to work for the body and there are significant decreases in postural muscle activity and in intervertebral disc pressure in the lumbar spine."[31]

DO

- ✓ Angle your elbows down to the keyboard, at around 120°.
- ✓ Use a chair with armrests.
- ✓ Position the keyboard so that the 'J' key is more than 12cm from the edge of the desk.
- ✓ Tilt your head downwards to look at the monitor.
- ✓ Angle the back of your chair at about 110°

DON'T

- ✗ Have the keyboard above your elbows.
- ✗ Use a wrist rest.
- ✗ Twist the shoulder out to move the mouse.
- ✗ Twist the wrist inwards to move the mouse.
- ✗ Use a lot of force when depressing keys.
- ✗ Sit with your back at a 90° angle to the chair.

Ways to click and type less

Autocorrect

You can use Microsoft Word's AutoCorrect feature to help you type less. Go to File, Options, Proofing, and then AutoCorrect Options. A window will pop up which has a 'replace' box and a 'with' box. By typing the shortcut (i.e. 'novb') into the first box and the full word (i.e. November) in the second box, then clicking add, you can add endless automatic shortcuts to Word. From then on, whenever you type 'novb' Word will automatically replace it with 'November', and you can do this for any word you find yourself having to type out regularly.

Shortkeys

ShortKeys goes beyond AutoCorrect, allowing users to specify a combination of keystrokes to serve as the shortcut. The user only needs to type a short sequence of keystrokes, before ShortKeys fills in the rest automatically with user-specified text (up to 3000 characters long). The advantage of ShortKeys is that it functions in all programs, which means that frequently-typed sentences and paragraphs can be easily entered in all applications. The user-defined shortcuts can be as long as 32 characters, and can include a prefix or suffix, such as ##, to avoid accidentally triggering replacement text. A free version of ShortKeys is available from www.shortkeys.com

Clickless software

Clickless software saves you from having to click the mouse. When you pause the mouse pointer for a short time over something on your computer screen, the software performs a click for you. This is particularly good if you find clicking the mouse aggravates your injury more than moving the mouse. A 30-day trial of clickless software can be downloaded from www.aerobicmouse.com (QuillNib). RSIGuard (*see below in 'Breaks'*) also has a clickless software feature.

Keyboard shortcuts

You probably already know some keyboard shortcuts like Ctrl-c and Ctrl-v for copying and pasting, but Microsoft Word has many other helpful shortcuts. To find them, press F1, search 'keyboard shortcuts' and click on 'Keyboard shortcuts for Microsoft Word on Windows'.

Mousing

Position

Make sure you're comfortable. You should be able to relax your shoulders and have your mouse close in to your body, **not** out to the side or up on top of your desk. Don't hold your wrist at an angle, or reach across the desk for your mouse - have it directly in front of your hand. You can buy a compact keyboard (without a numeric keypad) which leaves room to put the mouse in a good position.

Holding the mouse
Hold your mouse lightly and be as relaxed as you can. Have the cable pointing away from you and moving freely - make sure it's long enough. Click the buttons lightly, then relax your hand and try using two fingers to click. Unless your mouse is infrared, it's important to clean it regularly–you'll be surprised by how much better it works!

Choosing a mouse
Find one that fits your hand - move it around and practice with it to make sure it feels good. If you usually use the mouse with your left hand, get a mouse that is specially designed for left hand use. However, be careful about changing hands if one is injured - this may just lead to damage on the other side.

It's worth trying out a 'scroll-ball' mouse as this minimises dragging, the most dangerous mousing activity. Another option is to buy a **vertical/upright mouse** - this is the safest kind of mouse as it allows you to rest your arm on the desk in a more natural position.

Try using two mice
Many people with RSI finding that switching between a left-handed mouse and a right-handed mouse, one on each side of the computer, every five minutes or so, is a really good technique for minimising strain on the arms and shoulders. It may feel awkward at first but it will quickly become quite natural.

Breaks
Take breaks often - even short breaks help to reduce the risk of injury. If you have trouble remembering to take breaks, it's a good idea to get some break software. RSIGuard, available from www.rsiguard.com, is particularly good as it also includes clickless software (see above).

A lot of people find relaxation mini-breaks helpful; one major advantage is that the people around you won't notice them. To take a relaxation mini-break, sit in your chair, hands in your lap, and gradually focus your attention on different parts of your body. Firstly, move your focus from your head, to your neck, then to your shoulders, your elbows, your forearms and your wrists – relaxing each part of your body in turn.

Remember to vary the type of work you do and the position you sit in on a regular basis. This is one of the most important steps in avoiding injury. Set limits on how much time you spend using the mouse (break software can be useful here too).

Keep the blood flowing
Good circulation keeps your arms healthy. You can achieve this by getting regular exercise – try taking a brisk walk at lunchtime or before work. Wearing warm clothes (make sure they're not too tight) and cutting down on cigarettes and alcohol will help. As well, stand up regularly and move about: swing your arms, shrug your shoulders and jump up and down.

Stress
Stress causes increased heart rate, blood pressure and muscle activity and tension. The lower the muscle activity, the safer the user! It's really important not to be hurried and stressed when using a computer so try to relax – particularly when you're mousing.

Alternatives to mousing?
No alternative has been shown to be injury-free, but using a lightpen, a trackball or a tablet uses different muscles – and this means your usual mouse muscles are given a rest.

Computing by Voice

Voice-operated computing has developed significantly since it first emerged about 15 years ago. At that time, the software could only identify individual words and made a lot more mistakes than it does today. Nowadays, voice-operated computing actually works best when longer phrases and sentences are spoken and accuracy can approach 100%. There are many computer tasks that can be done by voice – you can dictate, punctuate, format, navigate, correct recognition errors, command the computer (either using built-in commands or custom macros), edit text, open applications and documents, write and manage emails, browse the web and edit spreadsheets.

Dragon NaturallySpeaking is the market leader in voice-recognition computing for PCs. While it is available for Macs, it doesn't work as well as it does on Windows. Dragon works best in Microsoft Word, Excel, Outlook and Internet Explorer. Another product you can use is Phillips SpeechLive.

There are four things to consider when trying to improve the performance of your voice-recognition software – the environment, the equipment, knowledge of how the software works and knowledge of the software's limitations.

Firstly, it's important to work in a fairly quiet environment. However, it's possible to use voice-recognition software in an open plan office environment, particularly if you have a very good quality microphone. The most likely background noise to interfere with the performance of the software is the sound of people around you talking.

The computer specification requirements of Dragon Naturally Speaking are quite high – so check them before you buy the software. The sound card also needs to be good quality – consider upgrading your sound card to something like Creative Labs Sound Blaster Live or Audigy. Alternatively, you may want to consider purchasing an external sound card that can plug into your USB port. Remember, that if your software appears to be performing well, there's no need to be concerned about these requirements.

The computer microphone is perhaps the most important piece of equipment. Features to look for in a microphone are a headset with noise-cancelling properties and an adjustable mouthpiece. Wireless microphones rarely equal the performance of a headset. You may need to buy a higher-quality microphone than the one that comes with the software.

Voice-recognition software works by picking up sound waves via the microphone in analogue format, which are then converted to digital format by the sound card. This is then compared to the software's vocabulary to produce text on the computer screen. The software uses a language model, which analyses the probability of a word occurring in speech – not only overall, but also in the context of other words. It also works on the statistical probability of two, three or even four words occurring together.

This is why you will get better recognition if you speak in longer phrases or sentences. For example, while the phrases 'whirled tour' and 'world tour' sound the same, the software will choose the latter because it's more common in speech. Remember, though, that the software tracks the language of each user individually - so if you're a person who frequently says 'four examples' but rarely says 'for example', over time the software will recognise this. Most importantly, it's the user correcting the errors the software makes that improves its accuracy most substantially.

It's also important to know the software's limitations. Having realistic expectations will prevent you from becoming frustrated. For people who are attempting to limit their physical use of the computer, be aware that it's not possible to use your voice for everything. For example, logging in must be done manually because the software cannot load until the computer is logged on. Also, a sound check must be carried out every day; this cannot be completed by voice alone.

There are also some tasks that are extremely tedious and inefficient to do by voice, such as performing spatial tasks in graphics programs.

It can also be challenging for new users to speak while they're thinking about what they want to write next, particularly when they're dictating complex documents. Some people adapt to voice-operated computing very easily, while others take longer – so be patient with yourself.

The process is often more difficult for people who were really competent with computers before their injury but now cannot use their hands for computing. Patience is definitely necessary when you're using voice-recognition software because correcting errors can be a very stop-start process, particularly for new users.

Unlike keyboarding, system error can occur up to 5% of the time, so, even if you do everything right, the software will still occasionally make mistakes. The process of proofreading is also different for documents that are 'written' by dictation because there will be no spelling errors in the traditional sense, and so to edit you must read for meaning.

Sound quality is obviously an important factor in helping you to get the best results out of voice-operated computing. While the microphone and computer sound card are two important components, the speaking style you use is also important. Gaining control over speech can often be a big challenge for new users because you need to speak in a very clear way (without 'ums' and 'ahs'). It's also really important to turn the microphone off when you aren't speaking; this prevents the software from interpreting background noise as speech, and also protects the microphone from damage and wear.

Speaking clearly and naturally is important. In fact, the software will recognise phrases better than individual words (this is particularly true of the most recent versions). Running words together or speaking too conversationally will lower accuracy. When giving commands, it's best to pause before the command and then say it as a clear phrase (without pausing midway through). As well, it's essential to perform an audio check every day to ensure that sound quality remains high.

Another thing to note is that the software recognises *words*, not letters, unless you give a specific command. So, if you say the letter 'p', this will be interpreted as 'pea'. People are often surprised by the fact that more technical and complicated words are often recognised faster than simple words – but this is because a word like 'for' is very common and sounds a lot like the words 'door', 'floor', 'or' and 'all'. Technical terms are often more unusual, more distinctive and longer, making recognition easier.

The best way to tell if your software is performing adequately is to note its accuracy and speed. Try dictating a passage of around 200 – 300 words and count the number of errors; if your speech is clear, you shouldn't have more than about five mistakes. If the number is higher, there are a number of things you can try:

- Correct your recognition errors. This is absolutely crucial. Use 'correct that' to teach the software more about your writing and speaking style and the words you're more likely to use. In time, this will lead to fewer errors.
- Customise the vocabulary. If there are names, places, objects or any other words that you use frequently which are not in the vocabulary, it's a good idea to add them. If a word you want to use is not in the vocabulary, the software has no chance of getting it right.
- Scan electronic documents to customise language model and vocabulary. This is a quick way to perform both the steps above – but just make sure the documents are written in the same style that you'll be dictating in!
- Do some longer training readings. If you do one or two of the longer training readings, this will

improve the ability of the software to recognise your particular speech patterns.

- Create custom commands (macros). In the 'Professional' edition of Dragon Naturally Speaking, macros let you add large chunks of text with a simple command. This is good for eliminating the time taken to dictate sign-offs, addresses, business names and other common sentences. It's also possible to create macros for commands such as inserting pictures or formatting.
- Try using the software in a quieter environment. This is the best way to see if background noise is having an impact on the software's accuracy.
- Be sure to close Dragon before logging off or shutting down. Failure to do this may result in the updates to your language model and speaking style not being saved.

For more help with Dragon NaturallySpeaking, download the user guide from www.nuance.com. This website also has a helpful discussion forum.

Our thanks go to Sue Woodward, Dragon trainer, for her help with this section.

Taking care of your voice

Most of us think of our voices as indestructible – a part of us that can't be damaged or destroyed. Yet we rely on two small muscles when using our voice, our vocal cords. Like other muscles, these can be damaged by overuse so it's important to take care when using voice-activated computing.

In fact, people who use their voice in their work often develop vocal problems. For example, 22% of teachers regularly experience voice problems; many singers have had to give up promising careers because their voice failed them and you may remember politician and Premier of New South Wales, Neville Wran. His voice was so tested by a sore throat during an election campaign that he required an operation and never sounded the same afterwards.

People who take up voice-operated computing can experience the same problems.

"When I first started voice-operated computing, I lost my voice a number of times as a result of overdoing it", says one RSI sufferer. Another member was using voice-operated computing in the days when you had to dictate one word at a time: "I began to suffer from intense headaches and jaw problems ... and was actually diagnosed as having an overuse injury of the jaw."

There are precautions you can take to minimise the risk of voice overuse. Firstly, good posture is just as important when using your voice as when using the rest of your body. One suggestion is to try dictating without looking at the monitor because this allows you to stand up, move around and reduce tension in your body.

Equally, you'll need to give your voice muscles a rest, just as you do with other muscles in your body. When you take up voice-operated computing, the muscles you work with are no longer resting when you go to a meeting, have lunch with friends, talk on the phone, or sing along with the radio. You'll need to plan rest breaks for your voice and build up dictation gradually, from maybe half an hour a day to a maximum of three hours a day.

It's also important to try to use your voice as naturally as you can. Some people adopt an unnaturally quiet voice when using a voice-operated computer, while others speak in a monotone; both of these are putting a strain on your voice. Try to vary your pitch and delivery in the same way that you would when speaking to a friend.

Voice-operated computing can be very stressful, especially when you're first learning to use it. Sometimes, the software seems to refuse to recognise practically anything you say and this can make you feel very frustrated. You need to develop strategies to deal with this; one member says she gives herself a break for a while and does something else. Other strategies include:

- getting extra tutorials in voice-operated computing to help improve your technique
- training the software in new vocabulary or any words it finds difficult to recognise
- doing some more training
- checking the audio levels
- checking that your microphone is properly positioned

Two things that your voice needs to operate well are warmth and lubrication. Your vocal cords need to be moist to work properly: this means that you'll need to drink plenty of **room temperature** water **before** you start working, and you need to keep drinking as you work. You may need to increase your intake of liquids if you're working in a very dry air-conditioned environment. Dehydrating substances like alcohol and caffeine should be avoided and smoking won't do your voice any good either.

Check with your doctor about medications you may be taking - some of these can have a dehydrating effect as well.

Other things to avoid include:

- coughing or clearing your throat (try sighing instead)
- yelling
- whispering
- trying to talk over noise
- slumping
- saying the same thing over and over again

Many people find that particular commands can strain their voice and macros can be helpful here.

Finally, don't be tempted to maintain the same work habits that contributed to your overuse injury when you switch over to voice-operated computing. Behaviour such as perfectionism, taking work too seriously, working to impossible deadlines without sufficient breaks and not making time to relax and exercise can all contribute to voice injury.

Writing

Writing by hand when you have RSI can be an awkward, painful task, but it's often preferable to using a keyboard. Here are some tips to help make it a bit easier.

Use the right pen

Cheap and tacky pens are everywhere—avoid them. Choose a pen that writes easily – we like the *Artline 'ErgoLine'* pen because it has a nice thick grip and requires very little pressure, as does the *Uniball 'Micro Deluxe'*. Most fountain pens are like this too. Pens with gel ink are generally easy to write with; don't bother with ballpoint pens.

Pen grips are available from newsagents and stationers and make a pen easier to hold (though you may need some help to put them on the pen in the first place). Another trick you can try is wrapping bubble wrap around the pen and securing it with tape or a rubber band.

Adapt your workspace

A slope-board, angled at about ten degrees, makes writing much easier because it minimises neck strain. Plenty of room to write on is important so clear a good space on your desk.

Adapt your writing style

One form of RSI, called focal dystonia, (otherwise known as writer's cramp) is caused by misfired signals in the brain that make your hand involuntarily cramp, making your writing painful and jerky.

One way to manage the problem is to write using your shoulder joint, rather than your wrist and fingers. Grip the pen lightly, and move your whole arm to create the letters. Write large letters and use large pads of paper because this requires less fine-motor control.

You can also try changing your grip. The following grip technique reduces the tension in the thumb, and balances the use of tendons crossing the wrist and small muscles in the hand:

- hold the pen between the index and middle finger
- bring the tips of the thumb, index, and middle finger together in the most extended position
- now, gently insert a pen, separating those fingertips

This is probably not the grip you'd normally use to hold a pen, but it's well-worth the patience and practice required to master it successfully.

Dr Hunter Fry, an Australian hand surgeon and authority on RSI, believes that most of us use a lot more force than necessary when we're writing. He offers the following experiment to demonstrate this:

1. holding the pen as lightly as possible with the grip described previously, write two or three words down slowly on a piece of paper (this will show you just how little muscular effort is required to move the pen)
2. remember that effort, and then compare the amount of muscular effort used after writing half a page in your normal way, writing as fast as possible

Dr Fry's rough calculation indicates that many writers would probably use a hundred times more muscle power than the amount actually needed.

Only write what you need to
One of the quirks of modern society is its excess of information. As such, it's important not to write down things that aren't that important, and restrict yourself to only noting down important information.

If you're a student, for example, only write down the relevant points in lectures, because lectures are supposed to be *listened* to. You don't need a record of every word that's said. If you restrict yourself to only writing down the important points, this will not only save your hand from unnecessary activity, you'll also develop important listening and memory skills and probably enjoy the lectures more too.

If you must take notes, a voice recorder (or dictaphone) can do it for you. Try and find one with buttons that are easy to operate.

When it's painful, avoid it

Even if you *can* write for prolonged periods, it's going to get painful eventually. Of course, when it's painful the best thing to do is avoid writing altogether. When writing becomes painful, try the following things:

- take breaks to allow your hand and arm muscles to relax
- use printed address labels when addressing envelopes so you don't have to write out addresses
- get other people to fill out forms for you

Other Ideas

Take a good look at your work area – is there enough room to work in and is the area free from clutter? If not, would an inclined surface help? If using a pen and paper or a handheld device is difficult, try some of these ideas for common activities.

Writing Letters and Cards:

- Write a progressive letter (do a little bit at a time) or photocopy a general letter for all your pen pals, adding a little extra to each to make it more personal.
- Send a card or postcard instead of a letter.
- For holiday seasons or celebrations, have pre-printed labels from your mailing list for repeated use and photocopy invitations rather than writing them.
- Make a telephone call instead.
- Try using pre-stamped envelopes; a self-inking stamp or address labels for your return address

and computer-generated bulk address labels for frequent addressees.

Diary / Planner:

- Get a large diary so that you can write in larger letters, which is often easier.
- Clip appointment reminder cards into your diary.
- Use abbreviations or codes rather than writing in full.

Note-taking:

- Use a voice-recorder.
- Consciously limit the amount of pen-holding and handwriting you do to reduce static load.
- Use a scribe.

Keeping a journal/diary

- Talk to others as a means of clarifying thoughts or problems.
- Use other methods to record your ideas and feelings (e.g. mind maps, dot points, drawing a picture of how you feel about something).

Lists

- Prepare master lists to photocopy. For example, list the main items you shop for on your shopping master list and highlight or tick items needed.
- Use fridge magnets with pre-written reminder messages on them, which will also stick to filing cabinets or white-boards.
- Set up a tickler file to help you stay organised.
- Set up reusable reminder cards that you can take with you or pin to a corkboard (e.g. blank business cards). For example, 'withdraw money', 'pay electricity bill', 'buy bus tickets'.

Paying bills and filling in forms:

- –   Set up direct debits by phone.
- –   Get help from friends, family or staff.
- –   If it's cost effective for you, take advantage of your bank's services such as regular cheque payments, telephone banking, ATMs, EFTPOS and direct debit.
- –   Use cash instead of cheques (post offices are agents for most essential services).

Additional Resources

Have a look at the 'Helping Hand' information sheets on our website www.rsi.org.au. These cover lots of tasks that are hard for people with RSI and we update them regularly.

CHAPTER 6
SPECIFIC CONDITIONS

Tennis Elbow

Lateral epicondylalgia (commonly known as 'tennis elbow') is one of the most common upper extremity musculoskeletal disorders. Researchers estimate that about 1–3% of the general population suffers from the condition, which affects the tendons on the outside of the elbow when the hand is palm-up.

It's a very painful condition which is aggravated by gripping and manipulating objects so things like picking up a cup of tea, unpacking shopping, and even shaking hands can be painful.

The reason it's called 'tennis elbow' is because of its very high prevalence in recreational tennis players - as many as 50% of people in this group will experience it in their lifetime. However, elite tennis players rarely experience tennis elbow. Work-related activities are one of the most common causes.

When researchers investigated a group of 60 people with lateral epicondylalgia to see what was likely to lead to a quicker recovery, they found that 80% of participants reported that they improved over a six-month period and 33% were completely recovered. [32]

Risk Factors
These researchers found that two features predicted a poor recovery very clearly: being a woman and having repetitive work duties, particularly if duties involved computers. The risk of symptoms was much higher amongst women using computers than men and the authors suggest that this may be due to less strength in the cervical and shoulder muscles in women. This, as well as their smaller stature, means

women need to use more musculoskeletal force when operating the keyboard and mouse.

This study suggests that even when overuse injuries are not caused by repetitive tasks, **computer work and other jobs which require repetitive movement may aggravate the condition and slow recovery**. For this reason, it's important to avoid any activities that cause you pain when you have an overuse injury, even if they didn't trigger the onset of your condition.

Treatment
So how is tennis elbow treated? Unfortunately, as with most overuse injuries, little research has been carried out into effective treatments. As a result, many of the guidelines you will come across are not evidence-based. Three of the most common treatments are steroid injections, physiotherapy and 'smart rest'. Recent research from the University of Queensland has shown that these different treatments have very different outcomes.

Cortisone Injections:

In the first three to six weeks, a steroid injection of prednisone resulted in the least pain and debilitation. However, after this short period, having a steroid injection actually predicted a slower recovery rate and a **much higher recurrence rate**—about 72% of people treated with steroid injections who felt fine at six weeks were experiencing the same symptoms again within a year.

Physiotherapy:
The most common physiotherapy technique used for this kind of injury involves a gentle and specific manipulation of the elbow, and people who received this treatment were also doing well at six weeks.

Smart Rest:

People in the 'wait and see' group of the study (who were just given advice on 'smart rest' strategies) did not do so well in the first six weeks but after about three months, they caught up with the physio group in terms of recovery rates. About 70–80% of the 'wait and see' group were fully recovered after a year.

Rest might be the best treatment for tennis elbow, but this does not mean putting your arm in a sling! If you rest the affected muscles completely, they will weaken because movement actually helps the rehabilitation process. This is where 'smart rest' comes in. **While common sense dictates that you avoid any activities that cause you pain, it's important to be as active as possible in other ways.** This speeds recovery.

Carpal Tunnel Syndrome (CTS)

The 'carpal tunnel' is like a rigid bracelet of bone and ligament inside your wrist. Through it run nine finger tendons, arteries, veins and the median nerve, which conducts messages from the brain through the arm to the thumb, forefinger, middle finger and ring finger. If the lining of this 'bracelet' becomes irritated and swollen, there's pressure on the median nerve, which impairs its ability to carry nerve impulses, and this then leads to carpal tunnel syndrome. Symptoms of CTS include pins and needles, tingling and numbness in the fingers, an inability to feel, dropping things, pain and soreness.

A little bit of history...
Dr George F. Phalen was one of the pioneers of carpal tunnel surgery and the modern understanding of carpal tunnel syndrome. He published a number of articles in support of a physical pathology for CTS. However, he also contended that CTS had no known cause. His main evidence for this assertion was that the majority of his patients were women.

Thus, a seemingly medical and scientific judgment about disease causation was based on a social perspective that

regarded males performing work in
heavy industry to be the type of patients
who could be judged legitimately to
engage in strenuous use of the hands.
Other work, whether cooking, typing,
sewing, or working in an office, was
relegated to the domain of 'women's
work', perceived as inherently less
demanding upon the hands and wrist.

Penny Kome, Wounded Workers: The
Politics of Musculoskeletal Injuries.[33]

Diagnosing Carpal Tunnel Syndrome

The diagnosis of carpal tunnel syndrome is not straightforward. It's relatively easy for doctors to determine that the median nerve is compressed, but whether it's compressed at the wrist is harder to decide. In the 'Wounded Workers' report published by the University of Toronto, Dr Susan MacKinnon is quoted as saying that people who keep their forearms in the palm-down position for long periods (i.e. when keying) can have a short and tight pronator teres muscle in the forearm [34]. This can compress the median nerve and mimic the symptoms of CTS.

Methods of diagnosing carpal tunnel syndrome include taking a detailed patient history, nerve conduction tests and tests of pain sensation and sensitivity to touch.

Do you have Carpal Tunnel Syndrome? Take this quick test

- Do you get tingling in at least two of the first four fingers?
- Are symptoms worse during the night or on awakening?
- Do the symptoms get better when you shake your hand?

If you answered yes to two of the questions, some experts say there's a 97% chance that you have CTS. The next step is to see your doctor, have nerve and muscle conduction tests and (if diagnosed) begin treatment.

Treatments for CTS
Steroid injections

An injection of cortico-steroids into the wrist area is a common treatment, and studies show that it's likely to give good short-term relief of symptoms. However, reliable long-term studies indicate that there's likely to be no benefit to these injections over a longer period (a year, for instance). This result is similar to studies into the outcomes for steroid injections in other overuse injuries.

Splinting

It's generally accepted these days that night-time splinting is the way to go, and for CTS, there's evidence that 'neutral-angle' splints are more effective than angle splints. One reliable study found that patients who wore their night-time splints six or seven nights a week experienced good symptom relief as well as good results on nerve conduction studies.[35]

Other Treatments

There are other treatments available that don't have as much well-documented evidence behind them, but they may be worth trying nonetheless. These include yoga and therapeutic ultrasound. Nerve and tendon gliding exercises could also be worth a try, though there's less evidence of effectiveness.

According to research, treatments that are likely to be ineffective for CTS include:

- low-level laser therapy
- magnets
- chiropractic
- NSAIDs
- diuretics
- vitamin B6

143

Unfortunately, quality research has not been carried out into the effectiveness of massage and osteopathic treatment, so we don't have scientific evidence about whether these work or not.

Surgery

Carpal tunnel surgery is considered to be a "relatively simple procedure".[36] To create more room in the carpal tunnel, the transverse carpal ligament is cut, thus releasing pressure on the median nerve. Sometimes scar tissue from the nerve and its lining is removed. Research indicates that surgery can be a highly effective treatment for carpal tunnel syndrome under the following conditions:

- an accurate diagnosis has been made
- both the diagnosing doctor and the operating surgeon have extensive experience with CTS
- there is early intervention – surgery within six months of diagnosis is much more effective than surgery after that period.
- after surgery, four to six weeks of recovery is required, during which you'll need to rest your arm.

Recent Research on Treatments for Carpal Tunnel Syndrome
CTS in rats

Carpal tunnel syndrome has been induced experimentally in rats through repetitive tasks. One important finding from this research is noteworthy: the limb that was *not used* in the task also showed signs of damage. The researchers suggest that "clinicians should examine the limb contralateral to the side of primary involvement (that is, they should look at the less-used arm)."

Findings of CTS signs and symptoms in the less-used limb should not be taken as evidence for malingering. Studies in this animal model suggest a possible underlying mechanism in which the local injury-inflammation cycle stimulates a systemic response that, in turn, renders *both* arms more susceptible to inflammation – even in the absence of obvious exposure or injury. These researchers say that treatments that might suppress a systemic inflammatory response, such as oral non-steroidal anti-inflammatory drugs or even aerobic exercise regimes, should be considered in cases where both arms are involved.

CHAPTER 7
WORKERS' COMPENSATION

So you have an overuse injury and you think your work caused it. What now?

Should I Apply for Workers' Compensation?

This can be quite a difficult decision and the answer depends on a number of personal and work factors. There are advantages and disadvantages in applying for workers compensation. The **advantages** include:

- payment for medical appointments, including specialists, treatments approved by your doctor, pharmaceuticals, transport to medical and therapeutic appointments, home help and help in the garden
- a degree of income replacement, which often declines over time
- your workplace may provide you with ergonomic aids, training in voice-operated computing, a more ergonomic work setup, different duties, or even assistance to do your current job

The possible **disadvantages** include:

- your claim may well be contested if it becomes long term
- income replacement can be inadequate in the longer term, depending on your state laws

- once you have applied for workers' compensation, you may be discriminated against in both your present workplace and future applications for work
- you may be involved in a legal case that stretches over years
- you may be unable to access long service leave or recreation leave while you're on a graduated return to work, which can be years
- the whole process can be very stressful

However, many people do access workers' compensation and have quite a positive experience. When making this decision, it's a good idea to look at what alternatives you have.

- Do you have accrued sick leave you could use?
- Do you have long service leave you could take?
- Would it be possible for you to go part-time in your present workplace, if necessary temporarily?
- Can you survive financially on a lower or no salary?
- Does your superannuation provider insure you against permanent disability?

If you find that workers' compensation is not helping you, you can drop your claim at any stage, although this may disadvantage you if you decide to apply again later. It would be a good idea to document your reasons for dropping your claim and send a copy to the insurer.

Remember, your rights and entitlements in workers' compensation vary between public and private insurers and also between states. It's worth finding out what you can expect by contacting your insurance provider anonymously before you make a claim, or having a look at your state's workers' compensation website.

If I Make a Claim, will I be Successful?

While there is a widespread perception that most workers' compensation claims are not successful, this is not true. Most claims are in fact successful initially. However, you may be successful in your initial application but find yourself under a lot of pressure to return to work before your injury is healed, or to scale up to full-time work before you're ready. Your claim may also be contested at a later stage.

How do I go about Making a Claim?

This is the usual process in applying for workers' compensation:

1. You're diagnosed by your doctor with an injury that is caused, or contributed to, by work
2. You ask your workers' compensation provider for a claim form and fill it in with your doctor
3. The provider makes a decision to accept or reject the claim
4. Your doctor may recommend that you take a certain amount of time away from work to recover and that when you return it's on a gradual basis: "a graduated return to work"
5. Your doctor will also recommend therapies to help you get better and the insurance company will pay for these (you can definitely suggest to your doctor which therapies you think will be helpful, using the information in this book). Your doctor may also recommend that you have someone to help you with your normal tasks at home in the house or in the garden. This will also be paid for by the insurance company.
6. If your time away from work is more than a few days, you will be allocated a rehabilitation provider. This may be from a private company which specialises in work injury cases. Some

of these companies are ethical and helpful, but they are under a lot of pressure from insurers to get you back to work fast and can, in turn, put a lot of pressure on you to achieve that. Some companies specialise in achieving a quick return to work and often the name of the company will give you a clue.

7.   When you return to work, the rehabilitation provider will liaise with your doctor, your therapist, you, and your employer and may help to redesign your workplace so that you can work safely.

The workers' compensation system tends to work better with relatively short-term injuries. So if you recover fairly quickly, workers' compensation can work well. However, with long-term chronic injuries – and unfortunately, this is what RSI can become – it doesn't always work so well.

When the system stops working for you, you do have other choices, and these may include:

- applying for disability retirement under your super scheme
- going to a lawyer and exploring your rights in the legal system
- working part-time
- applying for another job
- retraining for a job that you're able to do
- taking time away from work to recover, and then exploring your options

Workers' Compensation: Your Rights

You have the right to:

- change your rehabilitation provider
- choose your own doctor or therapist and to change them
- have a lawyer

- take someone with you to medico-legal interviews (a really good idea!)
- write a response to medico-legal reports
- leave the workers' compensation system
- apply for other positions at work
- ask for a different medico-legal practitioner

Getting More Information

Remember, your rights and entitlements in workers' compensation vary between public and private insurers, and also between states. It's worth finding out what you can expect, by contacting your insurance provider anonymously before you make a claim, or having a look at your state's workers' compensation website.

For information about your entitlements, the following websites are helpful:

Commonwealth: www.comcare.gov.au

QLD: www.worksafe.qld.gov.au

NSW: www.workcover.nsw.gov.au

SA: www.safework.sa.gov.au

ACT: www.accesscanberra.act.gov.au

WA: www.safetyline.wa.gov.au

NT: www.worksafe.nt.gov.au

VIC: www.workcover.vic.gov.au

The Medico-Legal Appointment

Over the course of your claim, you will be sent to medico-legal appointments arranged by your compensation insurer or your solicitor. The intention of these appointments is for the doctor to provide an independent opinion *to the insurer* on your condition – they will not tell *you* what they think or what you should do.

In practice, though, the insurer's medico-legal consultants will often try to prove that there is nothing wrong with you, or that your injury was not caused by work, and your solicitor's medico-legal consultants will be trying to prove that there **is**. So the medico-legal doctor may treat you politely but their report may not reflect the way your injury was discussed during the appointment.

> *I had an expectation that he would be fair. At the very least I expected what he said or implied in the consultation would be reflected in his report but it wasn't. There was a whole chunk of it left out.*

However, some medico-legal consultants have an understanding of RSI and are willing to support a person with RSI.

> *The first medico-legal doctor appointed by the insurance company was actually very nice. It seemed that he had a good understanding of RSI and his report was totally supportive of my claim.*

It's also possible that you will be sent to a medico-legal psychiatrist. This is not necessarily a threat. Many people with RSI feel overwhelmed and frustrated with the process they are going through and psychiatrists can pick up on this and support you.

Medico-Legal Consultants

Medico-legal appointments can be very unnerving. You're being sent to a doctor who is going to make a judgement on you and your injury and you may feel that the outcome of your insurance claim rests with them. This can make you feel vulnerable and anxious.

Further, medico-legal consultants will often not give anything away during the appointment. They may not give you any clues about what they are thinking.

> *I saw a medico-legal who was appointed by my solicitor. I was under the impression that he would be nicer than the others I had seen. But I left the appointment feeling that he didn't believe there was anything wrong with me. And then he wrote a report in my favour!*

> *One of the medico-legals appointed by the insurer was actually quite pleasant. He even showed some sympathy when I explained my symptoms. But his report said that there was nothing wrong with me.*

Unfortunately, **what they say in their report is largely out of your hands**. But you can take some control of the situation by knowing your rights and responsibilities. This will help you to feel more in control during the appointment.

Rights and Responsibilities

There are a number of guidelines set out by various groups in relation to medico-legal consultants' responsibilities.

The following is an outline of the Australian Medical Association's *Position Statement* on medico-legal appointments. Here are the key points:

- The medico-legal assessor's role is to provide an impartial opinion, not to treat the patient.

- The assessor should be courteous, sensitive and professional.
- The assessor should introduce him/herself, explain their specialty and their role.
- The assessor should explain all aspects of the assessment, particularly if it will be intrusive or involve undressing.
- The accompanying person should be informed not to take an active part and should not offer an opinion.
- Consideration should be given for a friend to accompany the patient. Ideally, the person should not be a family member.
- Consideration should be given for same-gender assessors.
- The assessor must obtain consent to begin, especially if it's intimate or will involve taking samples.
- The assessor should be aware that people may wish to record the assessment; however, talk to the insurer first.
- The assessor should not offer any advice or opinion on the claim or medical or surgical management. If they do have concerns, they should contact the person's treating medical practitioner.

The Appointment

If a medico-legal consultant appointed to you has a reputation for writing negative reports for people with RSI, ask to see someone else. Ring up your insurer and say something like, "I would prefer not to see Dr X, as he is well known for his negative attitude towards people with RSI."

There are a few medico-legal consultants who are rude and disrespectful, but these are the exceptions.

Some pointers to help you prepare:

- It's important that you turn up to the appointment. If you don't attend, the insurer can and will cancel your payments.
- Likewise, if you turn up but are not cooperative or 'non-compliant', your payments may be cancelled.
- Make the appointment for a time when you know you are likely to have symptoms, for example, straight after work. This means that there will be at least some physical evidence of your injury.
- Take three statements with you:
  o a brief medical history
  o a work history
  o your current employment information

If the medico-legal consultant has not read your file, they will at least have your written evidence in front of them. If you say "I'd like you to take this as evidence", they are legally obliged to do so. This also shows the medico-legal consultant that you know your rights and are not willing to be intimidated.

It may also be possible to take another specialist's report with you, if you have a copy of one that is in your favour. However, you might want to check with your solicitor about this. Depending on whether you're with a private or public insurer, reports may not be shown to the other side until negotiation of your claim starts.

It may be possible to ask your GP or solicitor to send you to a similar specialist around the same time as the medico-legal appointment. This will provide some back-up if the medico-legal report is negative.

Keep in mind that you want to create a good impression with the medico-legal consultant in order to establish a more equal relationship. Wear clothes that you feel good in. As well, speak clearly and concisely so that there is no room for misunderstanding.

It's a good idea to take someone to the appointment as a witness. If you want to do this, tell the insurer in advance so they can advise the consultant. If the consultant does not want a witness sitting in, ask for a different doctor.

Try to choose a witness who is not emotionally involved in the case, but is someone you trust.

The witness should just observe the consultation quietly and no more. It's a good idea for them to take notes.

If you can't take a witness, ask if you can take a small voice-recorder. While taped evidence may not stand up in court, it may encourage the medico-legal consultant to keep his/her behaviour in line. However, you do run the risk of establishing a rather hostile tone to the interview.

The medico-legal consultant will probably ask you questions about where your pain is, what it feels like and when it started. It will help if you think about these things before the appointment. It may be useful to write them down and take the notes with you. This will mean that you don't forget anything while you're at the appointment.

Cooperate with the medico-legal consultant. You can object to anything you don't think is appropriate, but you don't want to appear uncooperative as this will reflect badly on you. However, if something is causing pain or is inappropriate, tell them that you're in pain or not comfortable with their request. The doctor will need your consent to continue with that particular part of the examination. You have the right to be treated with respect and the doctor has a responsibility not to cause you pain without your consent.

The insurer's medico-legal consultant may search for information or try to force you to 'slip-up' by asking you personal questions that are not directly related to your injury. If a consultant does this, ask them to explain their request and why they think it's relevant to your injury. If you're not happy with their response, you do not have to answer the question. Relate answers about your emotional well-being to your condition if they are in fact connected, for example, "Yes, I do feel worried because I don't seem to be getting better and am in pain all the time."

Answer the medico-legal practitioner's questions concisely, but don't offer extra information. The doctor may allow periods of silence during which you're inclined to speak – don't! You may offer information that they don't need to know or can turn against you.

Public and private insurers work in different ways, so you may or may not receive copies of medico-legal reports requested by them. However, it's **always** worth asking for them.

If you do receive a copy and it's negative, you can ask your GP to write a rebuttal to be forwarded to the insurance company. This can sometimes help to convince the insurer to continue your payments.

Questions about the Legal Process

There always seem to be people on TV getting filmed by insurance providers – is this a frequent occurrence?
Surveillance doesn't happen that often, and providers—particularly government providers – have strict policies in place for how this may be done. An example can be found on Comcare's website www.comcare.gov.au/the_scheme/fraud which details Comcare's fraud policies.

I often see ads for lawyers that seem to say that I don't have to pay if I don't win – what does this really mean?
Generally, they will offer this service if they think you have a good chance of being successful. However, legal firms are businesses aiming to make a profit, so remember:

- The legal firm needs to recover its costs. If you decide to pull out of the case before completion, you may incur costs incurred so far.
- The legal firm will want to recover ALL of its costs from your settlement so be prepared and be aware of what costs are involved. Some costs, such as medical reports, may have to be paid *before* a settlement.
- Clarify with your solicitor at the beginning of the process what exactly you both consider to be a 'win'. Make sure you're clear about this, as you may have different expectations. You may actually be under pressure to accept as a 'win' an outcome that you don't see as a win.
- You should read through any contract very carefully

Where can I find court details of cases similar to mine?

A good source of legal case history is available online through the AUSTLII Database at www.austlii.edu.au, which gives detailed information on cases, including cases which have acted as precedents in decision-making.

CHAPTER 8
RETURNING TO WORK

Returning to Work

If you have been given some time off work in order to recover, thinking about a return to work can be daunting. It's a time when many people with RSI are unsure about themselves and their job and feel they have little control over their situation. In theory, the return to work process is meant to help you get back into work without aggravating your injury, but it doesn't always work that way!

Returning to work will involve some or all of the following people:

- your rehabilitation provider
- your employer and/or case manager
- your doctor
- you

Discussions between these people will determine your position, tasks and hours when you return to work. A timetable may be put forward outlining a return to work program and the steps involved. You and your employer are then expected to keep to this plan.

However, the return to work process does not always run smoothly. Many people feel they are pushed into going back to work before they have a chance to fully or even partially recover. They feel fearful about perhaps losing their job or about how others perceive their time off.

You just feel so compelled. I kept
thinking that I would lose my job if I

*didn't go back ... You don't want people
to think that you are taking off too much
time or not making a contribution. You
feel forced to maintain the same
standard as you would if you were not
injured.*

Many people with RSI feel they have little control
throughout this process. They agree to return-to-work plans
that are not ideal for them because of the pressure they're
under. They're unsure of what is happening to them and
don't feel that they can speak up.

*You are in a confused state of mind, you
don't really know what is happening to
you: if you are going to get better or
continue to get worse. The focus of your
energy is on the pain that you are in and
particularly if you haven't got support
structures around you and people being
assertive on your behalf, you just feel
like you are caught in a strong current
that you can't get out of.*

The most important thing for you to remember during this
time is that you do have a right to speak up and make
suggestions about what could help you stay at work. Keep
in touch with your doctor about how you are managing the
return to work and its effect on your health.

Knowing When You're Ready

How do you know when you're ready to return to work?
With so many people pushing you in all directions, it can be
difficult to work out what to do.

Your doctor will give you a certain amount of time off
work. This may be a week, a month, or any length of time
depending on how he/she perceives your situation. After

this time, unless extended by your doctor, you will be expected to return to work, possibly for reduced hours.

If you don't feel that this is enough time, you can, and should, ask for more time off. However, you need to understand that your doctor may be under pressure from the insurer or case manager to return you to work as soon as possible.

There will be a number of people involved with your RSI - your doctor, your rehabilitation provider and your employer or case manager. It's likely some of them will be pushing for you to return to work, even if you don't feel ready.

You need to be aware of how your recovery is progressing and how you feel physically and emotionally, in order to manage the process and get a good outcome.

You have to live in your body for the rest of your life: they don't. So it's vital that you have a chance to recover. The decisions made at this point can be a turning point: a return to health or, in the worst case, a long period of chronic pain.

So you need to have a clear understanding of your injury and pain in order to know if you're ready to return to work. Look at the following questions to help you to understand what stage you're at.

Your Symptoms

- Is there considerable pain even when resting?
- Is the pain stronger after certain tasks?
- Are there some tasks you can now do that you couldn't do when you were first injured?

How would these symptoms affect your working capacity?

- Could you return to your previous position?
- If not, could you take on some parts of the position?
- How many hours a day would you be able to work without hurting yourself?

How do these symptoms affect your day-to-day life?

- Can you undertake household chores such as washing, cooking and cleaning?
- Can you still undertake hobbies or other interests?
- Are you pressuring yourself into returning because you're afraid of losing your job? Or maybe you're worried about what others will think of you if you take more time off work? In general, do you feel that more time off work would be beneficial to your recovery?
- Try jotting down notes or speaking into a voice recorder to answer these questions. It's often easier to understand your thoughts if they are out in the open. You might even want to try answering these questions at different times.

It's vital that your doctor understands the level of your pain and your limitations. If you don't feel ready to return to work, *tell your doctor and explain why.* They need to know what you can and can't do. It's difficult for anyone who doesn't have RSI, including your doctor, to understand the kinds of limitations it places on your activities.

> *I wrote down everything that I thought was important in dot points – what I couldn't do, if I did this, that happened etc. I wish that I had done that at the beginning – because when I handed this to my doctor, I realised that he had no idea that I was at work trying to do a physically demanding job without the capacity to do it.*

The more clearly your doctor understands the situation, the more chance you have of recovering. Discuss with your doctor the options you have, be open to their suggestions and offer your own. Don't be afraid to speak up to others as well – your employer, your rehabilitation provider and even your family and friends.

161

Explaining what's happening to you can be difficult, but will help you get a clearer picture of your situation. Try it out on someone your trust first; this way you won't feel overwhelmed when you have to speak to doctors, case managers or rehabilitation providers.

Stay ahead by:

- Helping your doctor to understand your injury - write a list of things that are difficult or you can't do at all and why.
- Discussing your options and thoughts with your doctor and someone you trust. Aim to work at a level where your injury does not flare up.

Your Rehabilitation Provider

The insurer will appoint a rehabilitation provider. Their responsibilities include working out a suitable return-to-work plan and helping you to find new employment or training. The rehabilitation provider will:

- conduct an 'Initial Needs Assessment' for home and work to determine what help is required for you and start arranging it
- speak with your doctor to determine what you can and can't do to give them a clearer understanding of your work ability
- arrange a meeting with your employer or case manager, yourself and possibly your doctor to discuss a return-to-work plan – this is the first step in getting back to work
- help you to find other work options if you can't return to your pre-injury employment

Rehabilitation providers are generally in the difficult position of trying to keep everyone happy. This can be almost impossible because of the often conflicting needs of the different parties. The rehab provider is a 'middle man' between you and your employer. They are there to help you

AND get you back to work, which means keeping your employer and the insurance company happy too.

To get the most out of your rehabilitation provider:

- Be clear about what you can and can't do.
- Don't let them force you into a decision you aren't ready for.
- Speak to them about other job options and possible tasks you could do.
- Use your rehab provider as a 'middle man' if your employer or case manager is not keeping to the agreed plan.

Return to Work Plan

This plan is designed to manage your return to work and limit the amount of pressure placed on your injury.

When you negotiate your return-to-work plan, you need to take an active part. You may know of jobs or tasks at your workplace that you can do. For example, you could move into a training position or work on the telephone if you're provided with a headset. You may be able to do your old work if you have secretarial help for a few hours a day. With voice-operated software and some training, you may be able to work at a computer. A check-out operator found that she was able to work at the returns desk for four hours a day, even though she couldn't do her former work.

It's a good idea to brainstorm where you might be able to fit into your organisation, or whether you could do something useful with some extra equipment or some modifications. One woman we know moved to new work within her organisation as a trainer for several months after she returned to work – and recovered completely.

Your boss and your rehabilitation provider may also have some ideas. Be as flexible as you can while respecting your limitations.

Your return-to-work plan must be achievable. There is no point agreeing to a plan you know you can't achieve. So you should be prepared to argue your case if you need to. Only you know exactly what is right for you so speak up for yourself.

Returning to Work - the Initial Meeting

You can feel outnumbered at these meetings, so go prepared to stick up for yourself. You may be able to take a supporter – a union rep or a friend. Be open to others' suggestions but keep in mind that you're the person who has to work through the plan, so it must suit you. Don't be afraid to offer your own suggestions if theirs aren't right for you.

Your return-to-work plan will set out your work hours and days, as well as things such as work restrictions and breaks during the day. This plan will generally be approved and signed by all parties present at the meeting. This way, no one can claim that they didn't know what was required of them.

Keep in mind that if you're to work, for example, four hours per day - but need to take a break for 15 minutes every hour – you will actually be there for five hours.

The recommendations made in these reports should be adhered to by your insurer, employer, case manager and you.

Initial Needs Assessment

This report is conducted by your rehabilitation officer to determine the type of issues that need to be addressed and to set a goal for your return-to-work program. It will address the following issues:

- the history of the injury
- your difficulties with daily living
- any emotional issues
- your current situation and work restrictions
- recommendations – for example:
  - workstation assessment
  - home assessment
  - guidelines for the workplace

A home assessment will look at your home and family situation to determine if extra home help is needed. Recommendations will be about the amount and type of help required, e.g. housework and gardening.

Workstation Assessment

This assessment will look at your job and the difficulties you're having. It will set out the problems identified with your physical workstation and the adjustments that should be made. These could include different equipment, e.g. a telephone headset or voice-operated software.

Task and Work Practice Recommendations

This sets out the limitations and recommendations for work. It will state the number of hours to be worked, along with the restrictions that apply such as limitations to typing, pulling and lifting, as well as exercises, task rotation and any other conditions relating to your work situation.

Progress Report

A progress report will restate the goal of the program and set out progress to date. It's put together after your rehabilitation officer has met with you and discussed your current situation. It will cover any improvement or difficulties you're still having, but it doesn't provide any recommendations.

Case Closure Report

This report will state the outcome of the program, the services provided by the rehabilitation officer and the current situation. This is written when you no longer need a rehabilitation provider.

While at Work

Once you're back at work, you will need to follow through with the timetable and plans that have been set out. Be aware of how you're coping with the workload and tasks. If you're having problems, let your case manager or rehabilitation provider know.

Don't feel forced to work at the same pace you were working at before your injury. You may not be able to, and may aggravate your injury. When you first return, productivity is not the issue – the purpose is only to reintegrate you into the workforce. So, keep to the plan set out, or, if you find that it's too difficult to manage, ask for it to be revised.

In an ideal situation, any employee returning to work will have support from their manager and their colleagues and feel that the job is worthwhile. Successful return-to-work programs are those where the worker feels valued and has positive support from management and other employees. Unfortunately, this is not always the case. As one member said:

> *They said that I could collect money for the Christmas party and I was just so distraught. It was so humiliating. I felt that people thought that I was stupid.*

Most people don't have a good understanding of RSI and overuse injuries. Not all employers are unsupportive because they don't care. In many cases, people simply do not know how to handle the situation. They won't know how it affects you and the kinds of limitations it places on your ability to work.

There is no easy way to explain RSI to anyone else but it will help if you tell your employer how it affects you in the workplace and at home. You should aim to be clear and straightforward in your approach. Remain calm and talk about how RSI affects your ability to work and do household tasks. If you don't feel comfortable with this, ask your doctor to ring your employer and explain what you can and can't do.

You may not be capable of doing your old job and your employer may struggle to find suitable work for you. It's sometimes the case that they won't, or don't, take time to look carefully and deeply into the situation.

> *When I went back to work I was basically useless so it was as difficult for my employer as it was for me.*

It's very easy to blame your employer for not finding the right job or blame yourself for not being able to work. However, blame won't help you to achieve what you really want. If you're not satisfied with your job, try these:

- Ask around in the workplace, and find out if there are any jobs that need to be done – this could be helping other co-workers with a task, finishing off work they haven't been able to, or perhaps assisting someone who has too much work and needs some help.
- Approach your employer with a list of suggestions of jobs you feel capable of doing. Point out that you will be doing something productive and worthwhile.
- Point out to your boss that you want to work and are still capable of working. Say to your

employer "I would like to do ..." and "I am capable of doing ..." Be direct and clear in what you want to do and how you will go about it.

- If your boss does not listen or brushes off your suggestions, don't give up. Put your ideas in writing; talk to your rehab provider. You deserve to be treated with the same respect as any other employee.
- You might be able to suggest that they give you two weeks to prove that you can do a job or help in a certain area. At the end of that time, if either of you is unhappy you can reassess the situation.

You may find that you encounter some hostility in your return to work. Because people can't **see** RSI and don't know much about it, they may not understand your limitations.

> *I had taken on a new job part-time but a lot of my workmates didn't understand and there was a lot of impatience. You know – "why can't you do that job?", "the other girl used to do it".*

Your aim is to feel valued in the workplace. If you accept jobs that are below your capacity, your employer will not know that you're capable of more. So go ahead – make suggestions, give feedback and stay in touch with your boss!

Stay ahead by:

- communicating with others involved in the process
- having a clear idea of what you can and cannot do
- standing up for yourself

Your Rights and Responsibilities

Knowing your rights and responsibilities is part of staying in control of your RSI. Here are a few points to help:

- You can request a new rehabilitation provider if you feel that the one appointed is not helping you.
- You can look for new employment.
- You can speak up for yourself and request changes to working conditions, return-to-work plans or anything else you're unhappy about.
- You always have a choice either to sit back and take it or to stand up and ask for change.
- Be prepared for situations by knowing your rights and being clear about your physical and emotional condition.

Finally...

All of the above is not meant to imply that you're at fault in any way if you feel powerless and outgunned or if people treat your badly. Having a poorly-understood work injury like RSI can be very disempowering, and you may be operating in a legal framework that does not give you the support you need.

So what can you do? When you feel you have little power, allies can be a tremendous practical and emotional support. They can include:

- your doctor
- a psychologist
- work place counselling service
- professional counsellors
- your friends
- union representative
- OH&S representative
- your lawyer
- a paid advocate
- the RSI Association

An ally can:

- go to doctor's appointments with you
- accompany you to AAT hearings, your lawyer, or a medico-legal examination
- listen to you while you talk about what's happening to you
- let you know about new strategies to try or give you a different perspective on what's happening
- find other allies for you.

What if You Can't Return to your Previous Job?

Sometimes, going back to your pre-injury job isn't an option. Particularly in the private sector, some small workplaces simply do not have positions for an injured worker. Sometimes, you decide to move on to something else.

When people get RSI, some begin to question their careers and whether they really want to continue down the path they've been on. Other options may emerge because the one they were following is no longer possible.

> *I was put off work by my employer and after some time sitting around feeling depressed and unsure of my own abilities, I came across an advertisement for a course that sounded really interesting. After completing the course I realised that I had all these options in front of me that I hadn't seen before.*

Try to spend some time thinking about your current career:

- Do you actually like your job?
- Are there other careers that you have thought about?

- Do you think you're more suited to a different field?
- Are you in a position where you can take some time off and recover, then think about retraining?
- What does it really mean to you and your family to have a career that is hurting you?

CHAPTER 9

OVERUSE INJURIES AND EDUCATION

When you have RSI, furthering your education can provide you with direction and security. You will have a goal to work towards and know that you're enhancing your skills and knowledge. This is especially important if you have felt bored or depressed about your work situation.

> *I wanted some intellectual stimulation.*
> *My work had become extremely boring.*
> *They didn't have any work that didn't*
> *involve high-pressure keying ... my*
> *brain was screaming out for some food.*

Studying gives you a feeling that you're doing something worthwhile for yourself. It can give you independence, boost your confidence, and provide you with a sense of achievement. These are things you often lose when you have RSI.

> *(Going to university) was a non-*
> *judgemental activity done among people*
> *that were being nice to me and made me*
> *feel that I was a worthwhile person.*

Options for Study

There are a number of options to consider. You can try a course at a community centre or enrol in a correspondence course to get you started. You don't need to overwhelm yourself by jumping into university or TAFE if you don't want to. But you might find that you get swept along with learning!

I did a couple of correspondence courses before I made the decision to go to Uni. I was really enjoying the challenge and found that I wanted to learn more and more.

It's important to find a course that interests you. It should be something you're passionate about or something that you have always wanted to do. Don't worry about what you think you should be doing – think about what you *want* to do.

The Education Network of Australia website www.edna.edu.au is a gateway to information about studying in Australia. It provides useful information for people thinking about going back to study including lists of education centres.

The following is an outline of each of the study options. There are some website addresses included for further information. Otherwise, contact phone numbers and website addresses can be found on the EDNA website or in the phone book.

University
Universities offer a wide range of courses and options. You can attend full time, part time, or even complete a course by correspondence (see correspondence courses section).

The thought of going to university can be daunting, especially if you haven't studied for some time. However, universities offer a lot of help to new students. For example, most universities have an Academic Skills Program which runs short courses on topics such as essay writing and time management.

Universities also have an obligation to assist students with disabilities or injuries. There will be a disabilities officer on

173

campus whose purpose is to provide you with the help you need.

A disability officer can provide, among other things:

- note takers for lectures
- voice recorders
- extra time in exams to allow for rest periods
- help negotiating extended deadlines
- help typing up essays from a recording (this option is often dependent on funding)

Any information you provide to a disabilities officer is totally confidential. They cannot speak to anyone about your injury unless cleared by you. Likewise, you do not have to tell your lecturers or tutors about your injury.

It can, however, be very helpful to speak to lecturers, tutors or heads of department. Most of the time they are more than willing to help.

> *I was amazed at how helpful the Disabilities Officer was and how sympathetic my lecturers were. They were prepared to supply notes for the lectures and give me extended deadlines for essays.*

Speaking to lecturers or heads of department **before** a course begins can also be very helpful. They can give you an idea of the workload and how suitable the course would be for you. It also helps you to get an idea of their attitude towards RSI. Many are very sympathetic and will negotiate alternative options for assignments. You may, for example, be able to give a presentation instead of writing an essay.

Universities also offer student counselling services. Counselling services can help with a range of issues, from making decisions about courses to getting over obstacles such as fear and lack of self-confidence.

If you do decide to go to university, don't be afraid to contact the disabilities office, heads of department and counsellors to find out what they have to offer. They are there to help you.

TAFE

Like universities, they have disabilities officers to help you through the course. They also provide counselling services if you're having difficulties in any aspect of your course.

Distance Education

There are correspondence or distance education courses in just about everything and they can be a great way to get back into studying. They are open to everyone and generally do not have any pre-requisites.

An advantage of correspondence courses is that they often don't have strict time limits (except for university study). This means that you can complete the course at a comfortable pace.

Correspondence courses can be a stepping stone to further education. If you have been off work for some time or are considering university study, these courses can help you gain some confidence in your abilities or simply get you into the right frame of mind.

One drawback of correspondence courses is staying motivated. If you don't have strict time limits or other students around to provide encouragement, it can be difficult to get the work done. So it's especially important that you pick subject matter you're going to enjoy.

These are a couple of contacts:

- Open Universities Australia (OUA).OUA offers university study to anyone, regardless of age and tertiary qualifications. They have many courses from universities across Australia. You can complete a whole degree or just a couple of units. Their website is: www.open.edu.au
- Open Training and Education Network (OTEN). OTEN offers similar courses to TAFE. The courses offered have been pulled

together from a range of learning institutions with the advantage of completing the course by correspondence. These courses are more vocationally oriented than university degrees. Their website is: www.oten.tafensw.edu.au

Some universities also offer correspondences courses. Take a look at individual university websites for more information.

Adult/Community Education Centres

Adult and community education centres offer a range of short courses for only a couple of hours a week. Often they have courses such as time management that are useful before you start TAFE or university study.

These courses can be a stepping stone into further study. They offer courses in a wide range of subjects and the workload is generally quite light. These education centres often focus on courses for enjoyment rather than academic learning.

The Education Network of Australia has the names and locations of community education centres in all states.

Making Study Work for You

This section provides some practical advice to make the study process work more effectively.

Plan ahead

Before you undertake a course of study, contact the Disabilities Adviser at the institution where you plan to study – they have a lot of valuable advice and practical help to give.

You will receive a subject outline of each course during the first week. Compare your assignments and examinations timetables for each subject. You may need to contact lecturers and negotiate assignment times with them. If you're not comfortable doing this or find the lecturer unhelpful, contact the disabilities officer and they will be able to negotiate with the lecturer for you.

> *I'm doing a degree just one unit at a time. It feels slow compared with previous times I have studied, but I know it's all I can manage.*

Lectures and note-taking

Lectures can be difficult for people with overuse injuries. Sitting and writing for long periods of time may be painful. The disabilities officer may be able to provide you with a note-taker to attend your lectures with you. However, this does provide a problem with concentration for many people. If you don't have to take notes, your mind may wander!

Almost all lecturers these days upload their lecture slides onto the university learning portal. One way to cut note-taking is to download and print the slides beforehand, then you can simply highlight important points or make small notes in the margins. Some lecturers also upload a copy of the notes that they are reading from, which can often give you a really good summary of the lecture without having to take down any notes. Another option is to arrange with other students to copy their notes.

Some universities pay students in the class for detailed notes of the lectures, which are then passed on to people who don't have the ability to make notes themselves.

You could also try making very brief notes during the lecture, even one-word notes, to spark your memory. Then, as soon as possible after the lecture, make longer notes onto a voice recorder or voice-activated computer. This can be an effective way of recalling the material covered.

Actually, many students take more notes than are necessary during lectures – you really only need to record down the key points. In a way, RSI can help you with this. You can only write a limited amount so what you do take down has to be to the point.

Another option is to use a voice recorder during lectures but you'll need to get the lecturer's permission first.

Library Work

Find out from the information desk at the library what facilities are available to help students with writing difficulties. This might include an area where voice recorders can be used and where there are desk slopes, ergonomic chairs and assistance lifting books from high shelves. Access may be available to a voice-activated computer linked to the internet.

Assignments

Writing assignments presents a problem – and voice-activated software is a good option. It can be difficult to use at first but it does have significant advantages. You can see what you're writing as you write and can independently produce a document similar to that of other students.

Another option is working with a voice recorder. Depending on the lecturer, they may be prepared to accept assignments on tape or presented orally. But working orally is quite different to working on paper. It can be difficult to gain a clear understanding of your thoughts if they are not written down in front of you. If you do decide to try this method try using two recordings: use one for your outline and listen to it as you record your assignments onto the other.

Another option is to have your assignment typed up. This can be expensive if you have to hire a typist to do it for you. However, the university or TAFE may offer this service or you may be able to ask a friend or family member to help you.

Exams and Tests

You may need to make special arrangements for exams and tests, for example, extended writing time, rest breaks or an oral presentation. Contact the disabilities officer and they will tell you about the correct procedures and help with arrangements where necessary.

Some of the special exam procedures that have been successful in the past include: the use of ergonomic furniture and a computer, longer time for writing, regular breaks to move around, the use of a scribe and speaking from notes into a voice recorder. With all of these, you need to prepare ahead to make sure the arrangements will work smoothly on the day of the exam. For example, if you're using a voice recorder, will you have to supply it? Will there be a power connection or will you have to use batteries?

Laboratories and Field Trips
These can present special difficulties. It's essential that you discuss with your lecturer (and possibly the disabilities officer) how you can handle these activities. You may need some help from the lecturer, demonstrators and fellow students.

Further information and help

Contact the Disabilities or EEO Coordinator at the institutions you're considering attending.

CHAPTER 10
PREGNANCY AND PARENTING

Lisa's Parenting Experience

Lisa got RSI early in her career. She struggled with it before realising the extent of the problem but decided not to let it stop her having a child. She now has a two-year-old daughter and works part-time. While raising a child hasn't been easy, she has found solutions to many of the problems that arise.

I'd had RSI for about six years when my partner and I decided we wanted to have a child. At that time, in 2000, I was working full time and attending regular treatments to manage the pain. It was a difficult decision because we were both nervous about the kind of impact pregnancy and looking after a baby would have on my body.

I was 31 at the time and my biological urges had set in so I wasn't going to let RSI leave me with the regret of not having a child. I knew that looking after a child wouldn't be easy. I also knew I could work out ways to deal with problems that arose. It has proven to be an ongoing process and challenges arise all the time. But having a baby is great fun and she reminds me of what is important in life.

During the first trimester of my pregnancy, I was worried about my body's ability to carry a child. I felt because I had one illness something else would go wrong. It took a couple of months to realise that my body could cope just as well as anyone else's and after that I didn't worry so much. Being pregnant turned out to be a lovely feeling and I had such a positive attitude towards my body. I was producing another person!

The pregnancy was like a holiday from RSI. My pain levels were the lowest they had ever been, I guess it was because of all the hormones. The little pain I did have I could manage through heat, stretching and walking in the pool to keep mobile.

I couldn't have the full range of treatments because of the pregnancy, but these three were enough to get me through.

Throughout the pregnancy, there was a lot to think about, and organisation was very important. My partner and I had to anticipate the problems that might arise and how we would cope so we gathered as much information as we could. We read everything we could find and spoke to other people with RSI who'd had children to learn how they coped. We also found community resources and services we could use, such as community nurses.

There were a lot of practical things we had to consider. Finding the easiest options, such as using disposable nappies and finding the highest cot, high chair and change table (so I wouldn't have to lift so far) were big considerations. The options weren't always cheap, though we found that we could invent solutions too. For example, we raised the height of the cot by taping together several Yellow Pages to put under each leg.

The labour and birth experience were challenging because there were only a few positions I could use without aggravating my neck or arms. The constant stress and tension didn't help either, but I got through it. The biggest shock though, as it's for all new parents, was the complete dependence and demands of a newborn baby. I had no idea how hard it was to look after a baby, let alone with an injury. Broken sleep, coping with breastfeeding, settling the baby without rocking or patting her and being able to get to treatments were the biggest challenges.

Broken sleep was hard because it's like a form of torture. It affects your ability to think clearly, and, with chronic pain, your ability to rest and heal at the end of each day. My stress levels and the soreness of my arms increased dramatically and some days I would just be sobbing because there was nothing I could do to ease it. Nor was there any

181

way around it. I had to get up and feed her, no one else could do it.

I found relaxation techniques helped when I was trying to get back to sleep and I took every opportunity to sleep while my daughter was sleeping. My partner and I attended the sleep clinic for advice on techniques to get her to sleep longer and wake less during the night. This helped with her sleep time, but getting her to sleep was particularly difficult for both of us. I couldn't rock her or pat her to sleep so I had to put her down and let her cry which made me very sad. Taking her for a walk in the stroller helped get her to sleep while she was small.

Breastfeeding wasn't easy either. I had difficulty holding her for long periods but I found a number of things to help me. A lactation consultant came to the house to show me the best way to position my daughter when I fed her so I was putting as little strain as possible on my body. This was really helpful because I was feeding eight times a day and had to be able to sustain this. I also learnt how much time was necessary to feed her and how I could reduce the amount of time I was spending. One of the best purchases I made was a special breastfeeding pillow that wrapped around my waist so I didn't have to use my arms at all. I took this everywhere, even to shopping centres.

Getting to appointments for myself and my daughter was a struggle in the beginning. I had a community nurse come to visit me at home for the first couple of months which helped but, I had to take her to appointments for my RSI and this was hard. Just moving her around was difficult when I couldn't carry her for long periods. I did find a massage therapist who came to the house which was a huge relief. I also learnt to give self-treatments like baths and stretching when I got sore.

Some of the difficulties do take the edge off having a baby because you're always thinking about the strain. Seeing other mums settling their babies and carrying them around was hard at times too. But at the same time having a child is an amazing experience. She is two now and there is so much laughter around the house that I often don't have time to worry about being in pain. The reality is that there is a lot of happiness and also a layer of complexity.

Each stage has difficulties, though I think it gets better every six months. Now that she is two she doesn't need to be picked up as much as she did when she was 18 months old. I can encourage her to do a lot more for herself now, which is good. I also think that she crawled and walked early because I encouraged her to do these things as quickly as possible!

Inventing and changing is constant. Even now I have to stand back and think about changes that can be made. For example, I recently asked myself – does she still need to use the high chair? I decided that she was ready to use the kids' table and chairs I had bought, which means that I don't have to lift her into the high chair anymore. I look at each activity and ask myself 'is this the best way?' If I decide it's not, I find or invent another way.

My partner is very important to me, he has been so accommodating and supportive. There has always been the extra pressure and the physical load on him has been much greater. From the beginning, there have been certain things I couldn't do, such as bathing our daughter or chopping vegetables. We have different roles and our daughter has learnt this too. She knows that mummy can't play certain games that daddy can, and she knows that mummy gives hugs on the floor and daddy doesn't. She copes well with this. I think children just adapt to what you teach them.

Going back to part-time work was, at first, a challenge. Now I think it helps me. It's easier with my daughter in childcare so I can go to treatments without having to take her with me. It also helps to create a nice balance for me. I alternate days at work and home so that I can alternate the types of activities I am doing.

Since she was born I have also had to set rules for the overall management of my RSI. This means only going out once a day, carrying her as little as is absolutely necessary, and ensuring that things are within easy reach. Learning to say no to her has been important also, but very hard, especially now that she is learning to talk back!

I have had two flare-ups over the past year which have forced me to take four or five weeks off work. Both times it was because my daughter was sick and I had to break my own rules. At those times I had to hold her more than I knew I should because I had no choice – she was ill and needed comfort. There are also times that I have to put strain on my arms by just catching my daughter to stop her falling and that sort of thing. These are things you just have to do with a child.

I don't work full days because my threshold is almost reached through other activities. My managers and most of my colleagues are understanding. I try to be very clear and upfront with my managers about what I can and can't do. I also try to give them as much room to move as possible and do as much as I can. It's a two-way thing, I can't just demand they accommodate me because there is work to be done and other people to think about. There has to be communication both ways and as a result people tend to be supportive and respectful of my situation.

I believe something happens to everyone in their life. I was young when RSI happened to me and there have been some benefits. I am kinder to myself these days and take much better care of myself. I am far more assertive than I used to be and it's because I believe I'm worth it now. I consider these to be good things that have come from my RSI.

Life is much less predictable than I thought it was before RSI and I now focus on the journey rather than the destination. These days I think about how, or even if, I am going to get there and ask what the rush is anyway. For the moment I am just focused on raising my daughter. I'm not negative about my work but it's not my priority. The only doubt I have is whether or not I will have any more children. My partner and I will have to decide that in the future when our daughter gets a little older.

My advice to anyone with RSI wanting to have a baby is that it's achievable, though it's not easy. However, while it's important to focus on getting the 'mechanics' of taking care of a child, the joy of being a mother – the joy of creating your child, nurturing your child, taking care of their emotional needs, laughing with your child and loving your child – is wonderful. During the times it does get hard, I found this quote has helped me:

When the heart weeps for what is lost,
the spirit laughs for what is found.

A Sufi Aphorism

Our book **"Pregnancy and Parenting"** has lots of useful information on products, strategies and solutions. It can be found on our website www.rsi.org.au

---

REFERENCES

Chapter 1

[1] Brennan, P. (1985) *RSI: Explorer's Guidebook*, Primavera, Sydney.

[2] The Australian OH&S Commission (1986) Draft Model Code of Practice for RSI Prevention and Management.

[3] Comcare (1997) Report into the incidence of Occupational Overuse Syndrome.

[4] For example, Holmes, B. (1999) 'The Strain is in the brain', *New Scientist,* Vol 162.

[5] Rosenman, M. (2000). Journal of Occupational and Environmental Medicine # 42, Vol 1.

[6] Arndt, P. (1986) *RSI Explained*, N.S. Hudson Publishing Services, Victoria.

[7] Arndt, P. (1986) *RSI Explained*, N.S. Hudson Publishing Services, Victoria.

[8] Pascarelli, E. & Quilter D. (1994) *Repetitive Strain Injury: A Computer User's Guide*, John Wiley & Sons Inc. USA.

[9] Quilter, D. (1998) *The Repetitive Strain Injury Recovery Book*, Walker Publishing Company, USA.

Chapter 2

[10] Carnes, D., Homer, K., Underwood M., Pincus T., Rahman A. & Taylor S J C. (2013) 'Pain management for chronic musculoskeletal conditions: the development of an evidence-based and theory-informed pain self-management course' *British Medical Journal.*

Chapter 3

[11] Reid, J., Ewan, C., Lowy, E. (1991). 'Pilgrimage of Pain: the Illness Experiences of Women with Repetition Strain Injury and their Search for Credibility.' *Social Science and Medicine* 32 (5), 601-612.

[12] Arksey, H. Sloper, P. (1999). 'Disputed Diagnoses: the Cases of RSI and Childhood Cancer' *Social Science and Medicine* 49 (4), 483-497.

[13] Konijnenberg, H. A., de Wildge, N. S., Gerritsen, A. A., van Tulder, M. W., & de Vet, H. C. (2001). 'Conservative treatment for repetitive strain injury.' *Scandinavian Journal of Work and Environmental Health, 27,* 299-310.

[14] Malliaras, P., Rodriguez Palomino, J. & Barton, C. J. (2018). 'Infographic. Achilles and Patellar Tendinopathy Rehabilitation: Strive to Implement Loading Principles not Recipes' *British Journal of Sports Medicine*

[15] Snedeker, J. G. & Foolen, J. (2017). 'Tendon Injury Repair- a Perspective on the Basic Mechanisms of Tendon Disease and Future Clinical Therapy' *ScienceDirect* Volume 63, 18-36.

[16] Vickers, A. J., Cronin, A. M., Maschino, A. C., Lewith, G., MacPhereson, H., Foster, N. E., Sherman,, K. J., Witt, C. M., & Linde, K. (2012). 'Acupuncture for Chronic Pain: Individual Patient Data Meta-Analysis.' *Archives of internal medicine*, 172(19), 1444-1453.

[17] Deare, J. C., Zheng, Z., Xue, C. C. L., Liu, J. P., Shang, J., Scott, S. W., & Littlejohn, G. (2013). 'Acupuncture for treating fibromyalgia.' *Cochrane Muscle Group.*

[18] Little, P., Lewith, G., Webley, F., Evans, M., Beattie, A., Middleton, K., Barnett, J., Ballard, K., Oxford, F., Smith, P., Yardley, L., Hollinghurst, S., & Sharp, D. (2008). 'Randomised controlled trial of Alexander technique lessons, exercise, and massage (ATEAM) for chronic and recurrent back pain.' *British Medical Journal*, 337.

[19] Huisstede, B. M., Gebremariam, L., Van Der Sande, R., Hay, E. M., & Koes, B. W. (2011). 'Evidence for

effectiveness of extracorporal shock-wave therapy (eswt) to treat cacific and non-calcific rotator cuff tendinosis – a systematic review.' *Journal of Manual Therapy*, 16(5), 419-433.

[20] Lundblad, I., Elert, J., & Gerdle, B. (1999). 'Randomised controlled trial of physiotherapy and feldenkrais interventions in female workers with neck-shoulder complaints.' *Journal of Occupational Rehabilitation,* 9, 179-194.

[21] Kim, T. H., Cha, R. L., Choi, T. Y. & Lee, M. S. (2012). 'Intramuscular Stimulation Therapy for Healthcare: a Systematic Review of Randomised Controlled Trials'. *British Medical Journal,* 30 (4), 286-290

[22] Fernandez-de-las-Penas, C., Cleland, J., Palacios-Cena, M., Fuensalida-Novo, S., Pareja, J. A. & Alonso-Blanco, C. (2017). 'The Effectiveness of Manual Therapy Versus Surgery on Self-reported Function, Cervical Range of Motion , and Pinch Grip Force in Carpal Tunnel Syndrome: A Randomized Clinical Trial' *Journal of Orthopaedic & Sports Physical Therapy* 47 (3), 151-161

[23] Loew, L. M., Brosseau, L., Tugwell, P., Wells, G. A., Welch, V., Shea, B., Poitras, S., De Angelis, G., & Rahman, P. (2014). 'Deep transverse friction massage for the treatment of lateral elbow or lateral knee tendinitis.' *Cochrane Musculoskeletal Group, 11.*

[24] Brossea, L., Wells, G.A., Tugwell, P., Casimiro, L., Novikov, M., Loew, L, Sredoc, D., Clement, S., Gravelle, A., Hua, K., Kresic, D., Lakic, A., Menard, G., Cote, P., Leblanc, G., Sonier, M, Cloutier, A., McEwan, J., Poitras, S., Furlan, A., Gross, A., Dryden, T., Muckenheim, R., Cote, R., Pare, V., Rouhani, A., Leonard, G., Finestone, H.M., Laferriere, L., Dagenais, S., De Angelis, G., Cohoon, C. Ottawa. (2012). 'Panel evidence-based clinical practice guidelines on therapeutic massage for neck pain.' *Journal of Bodywork and Movement Therapies,* 16, 300-325.

[25] Moraes, V. Y., Lenza, M., Tamakoi, M. J., Faloppa, F., & Belloti, J. C. (2013). 'Platelet-rich therapies for musculoskeletal soft tissue injuries.' *Cochrane Database Systematic Review.*

[26] Andia, I., Latorre, .M., Gomex, M. C., Burgos-Alonso, N., Abate, M., & Maffulli, N. (2014). Platelet-rich plasma in the conservative treatment of painful tendinopathy: a systematic review and meta-analysis of controlled studies. *British Medical Bulletin, 110, 99-115.*

[27] S de Jonge, & RJ de Vos. (2011). 'Platelet rich plasma for Chronic Achilles tendinopathy: a double-blind randomised controlled trial with one year follow up.' *Brittish Journal of Sports Medicine, 45.*

[28] Petrella, Cogliano, Decaria , Mohamed and Lee. (2010) 'Management of Tennis Elbow with Sodium Hyaluronate Periarticular injections' *Sports Medicine,Arthroscopy,Rehabilitation,Therapy &Technology* Volume 2

Chapter 4

[29] 'Natural first-aid' (2007) *Choice magazine online:* http://choice.com.au/viewArticleAsOnePage.aspx?id=1055 31

Chapter 5

[30] Lorig, K. & Fries, J. (2000) The Arthritis Helpbook: A Tested Self-Management Program for Coping with Arthritis and Fibromyalgia, 5th Ed, Da Capo Press USA.

[31] http://ergo.human.cornell.edu/ergoguide.html, Marcus, M., Gerr F., et al, (2002) "A prospective study of computer users: II. Postural risk factors of Musculoskeletal symptoms

and disorders*" American Journal of Industrial Medicine,*
41:236-249

Chapter 6

[32] Waugh, E., Jaglal, S. & Davis, A. (2004). 'Computer use associated with poor long-term prognosis of conservatively managed lateral epicondylalgia'. *Journal of Orthopaedic and Sports Physical Therapy, 34,* 770-780.

[33] Kome, P. (1998) 'Wounded workers: The politics of musculoskeletal injuries', University of Toronto, Canada.

[34] Kome, P. (1998) 'Wounded workers: The politics of musculoskeletal injuries', University of Toronto, Canada.

[35] Nobuta, S., Sato, K., Nakagawa, T., Hatori, M. & Itoi, E. (2008) 'Effects of Wrist Splinting for Carpal Tunnel Syndrome and Motor Nerve Conduction Measurements', *Upsala Journal of Medical Sciences*, 113:2, 181-192.

[36] Pascarelli, E. & Quilter D. (1994) '*Repetitive Strain Injury: A Computer User's Guide*', John Wiley & Sons Inc. USA.

Lightning Source UK Ltd.
Milton Keynes UK
UKHW012358071220
374785UK00004B/1153